"A recognized expert in abuse treatment, Libby Schmanke offers a beautifully written text [...] with substance use problems. Schmanke's thoughtfully presented case studies, collected and analyzed during decades of clinical and academic practice, inform theoretical constructs, clinical applications, and art-based interventions; this book is a must-read for art therapists, related professionals, and graduate students."

—*Gaelynn P. Wolf Bordonaro, Ph.D., ATR-BC, Professor and Director, Emporia State University Art Therapy Program and Board of Directors, American Art Therapy Association*

"Drawing extensively upon substantial literature and her own personal, professional, and clinical experiences, Libby Schmanke has provided what I strongly believe will be the quintessential text on art therapy in treating people with alcohol and substance addictions. From theories to assessments to interventions, Schmanke has confirmed the power that art has in treating, supporting, and empowering these oft-stigmatized, vulnerable people."

—*Dave Gussak, PhD, ATR-BC, Florida State University, Professor, Art Therapy/Chair, Department of Art Education*

"This is the book I wished had existed when I started as an art therapist in addictions thirty years ago. A highly experienced practitioner shows how contemporary biopsychosocial-based theory can be grounded in the real-world complexities of practice. I learned new things here and my recommendation is whether you are new or already working in this field, read this book."

—*Dr. Neil Springham, Consultant Grade Art Therapist, Oxleas NHS Foundation Trust, UK*

"Rich in content and thoughtfully presented, *Art Therapy and Substance Abuse* will fast become the go-to book for clinicians, educators, and students working with the population. A seasoned clinician and gifted author, Libby Schmanke has succeeded in capturing the art therapy and substance abuse field with her comprehensive, contemporary, inspirational, and practical text."

—*Holly Feen-Calligan, Ph.D., ATR-BC, Associate Professor and Coordinator, Art Therapy Program, Wayne State University, USA*

Art Therapy and Substance Abuse

of related interest

Music Therapy and Addictions
Edited by David Aldridge and Jörg Fachner
ISBN 978 1 84905 012 8
eISBN 978 0 85700 294 5

Tackling Addiction
Pathways to Recovery
Edited by Rowdy Yates and Margaret S. Malloch
ISBN 978 1 84905 017 3
eISBN 978 0 85700 369 0

Drug Addiction and Families
Marina Barnard
ISBN 978 1 84310 403 2
eISBN 978 1 84642 565 3

Complicated Grief, Attachment, and Art Therapy
Theory, Treatment, and 14 Ready-to-Use Protocols
Edited by Briana MacWilliam
ISBN 978 1 78592 738 6
eISBN 978 1 78450 458 8

Drawing from Within
Using Art to Treat Eating Disorders
Lisa D. Hinz
ISBN 978 1 84310 822 1
eISBN 978 1 84642 543 1

ART THERAPY AND SUBSTANCE ABUSE

Enabling Recovery from Alcohol and Other Drug Addiction

LIBBY SCHMANKE

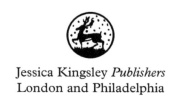

Jessica Kingsley *Publishers*
London and Philadelphia

The Twelve Steps are reprinted with permission of Alcoholics Anonymous World Services, Inc. ("AAWS"). Permission to reprint the Twelve Steps does not mean that AAWS has reviewed or approved the contents of this publication, or that AA necessarily agrees with the views expressed herein. AA is a program of recovery from alcoholism only—use of the Twelve Steps in connection with programs and activities which are patterned after AA, but which address other problems, or in any other non-AA context, does not imply otherwise.

First published in 2017
by Jessica Kingsley Publishers
73 Collier Street
London N1 9BE, UK
and
400 Market Street, Suite 400
Philadelphia, PA 19106, USA

www.jkp.com

Copyright © Libby Schmanke 2017

Front cover image source: Libby Schmanke

All rights reserved. No part of this publication may be reproduced in any material form (including photocopying, storing in any medium by electronic means or transmitting) without the written permission of the copyright owner except in accordance with the provisions of the law or under terms of a licence issued in the UK by the Copyright Licensing Agency Ltd. www.cla.co.uk or in overseas territories by the relevant reproduction rights organisation, for details see www.ifrro.org. Applications for the copyright owner's written permission to reproduce any part of this publication should be addressed to the publisher.

Warning: The doing of an unauthorised act in relation to a copyright work may result in both a civil claim for damages and criminal prosecution.

Library of Congress Cataloging in Publication Data
Title: Art therapy and substance abuse : enabling recovery from alcohol and other drug addiction / Libby Schmanke.
Description: London ; Philadelphia : Jessica Kingsley Publishers, 2017. | Includes bibliographical references and index.
Identifiers: LCCN 2017023164 | ISBN 9781849057349 (alk. paper)
Subjects: LCSH: Substance abuse--Treatment. | Arts--Therapeutic use.
Classification: LCC RC564 .S3243 2017 | DDC 362.29--dc23
LC record available at https://lccn.loc.gov/2017023164

British Library Cataloguing in Publication Data
A CIP catalogue record for this book is available from the British Library

ISBN 978 1 84905 734 9
eISBN 978 1 78450 118 1

Printed and bound in the United States

Contents

	ACKNOWLEDGEMENTS	7
	PREFACE: A STORY	9
	Introduction	17
1.	Findings in the Art Therapy Literature	22
2.	Substance Abuse Theory and Drugs of Abuse	43
3.	Incorporating Art Therapy into Substance Abuse Treatment Programming	63
4.	Assessment	87
5.	Group Work	109
6.	Feelings and Trauma	129
7.	Spirituality	150
8.	Diversity and Special Populations	170
9.	Families in Crisis and in Recovery	191
	APPENDIX A: SELECTED TECHNIQUES AND ACTIVITIES	211
	APPENDIX B: RESOURCES ABOUT SUBSTANCE ABUSE	227
	REFERENCES	231
	AUTHOR NOTE	244
	SUBJECT INDEX	245
	AUTHOR INDEX	251

Acknowledgements

I deeply acknowledge the many people seeking recovery with whom I have worked over the years. Whether you appeared on your own seeking help or were somehow coerced into treatment, I learned from each of you and feel honored to have had a place in your story. Thank you for bringing meaning to my life.

To Dr Gaelynn Wolf Bordonaro and Jessica Stallings, my faculty colleagues in the art therapy graduate program at Emporia State University (ESU), Kansas: I am so grateful to have such dedicated, positive-thinking, and supportive friends! Our satisfying hard work together over the last decade has solidified our 45-year-old master's program, and I always look forward to the rare times when we can relax and enjoy each other's company.

To current and former art therapy students, and in particular to Alison Boughn, Samantha Brandt, Michael Chavez, Valarie Colgate, Anna Davis, Kasen Keller, Raven Milam, Danielle Naeger, and Leslie Woodruff: your individual contributions, whether of a directive, illustration, or typing and formatting, are truly appreciated. Many other students also shared wonderful ideas for directives, but there was not room—maybe we should make a new book!

To Dr Ken Weaver, formerly our department chair and now the dean of our college: you have inspired me since I first arrived at ESU as a student. Your joy in all things academic was obvious; your ability to make writing and research seem fun and rewarding was a gift to those around you and has inspired my teaching. To Dr David Gussak, friend and once my graduate faculty advisor, who made me realize that learning to write well is a lifelong endeavor: thank you for supporting me and my professional development as an art therapist. The semi-colons are for you!

I appreciate people who work hard to make special places. This book would never have been written if not for my hideouts at the remarkable Topeka and Shawnee County Public Library, winner (over nearly 10,000 others) of the 2016 North American Library of the Year award; and at the cozy and peaceful Emporia Super 8 hotel, kept so fresh and quiet by manager Nimish Bhakta, his family, and staff.

I am ever grateful to Roger, my life partner of 40 years and counting: thank you, for always being there for me. I couldn't have had such an amazing life without you! And Rachel, dear daughter: you are already a beautiful person, and as you enter your career in criminal justice, I see a deeper transformation within you. I know that you will excel at helping others on the journey, and that you will find fulfillment in what you do.

My own identity, first and always, has been of an artist and a student, formal or otherwise. During the decade of my 20s, I was someone whose life revolved around alcohol and cocaine; beginning in 1986, I became a person in recovery; then a substance abuse counselor and program administrator; and finally, an art therapist and educator. The dream career I predicted for myself as a child was to write and illustrate books. I am grateful to Jessica Kingsley Publishers for inviting me to write this book, for allowing me to include so many color images, and approving my illustration for the cover. It has been exciting to have the opportunity to integrate some of my life learnings into this project, whereby I hope to "pass it on."

Preface

A Story

In remembrance of art therapy pioneer and my mentor, Robert Ault, for whom it was all about the art and the stories, this introduction is a story. It tells of a strong woman I will call Irene and her breakthrough in communication via an art task, and of the related events that led me to become an art therapist. This story also references the experience of people with trauma and substance abuse issues who have been criminalized.

Early in the 1990s, when sentencing for drug convictions was particularly harsh and open-ended, Irene was incarcerated in the state women's prison where I was working as an addictions counselor. She had been a low-level street drug peddler and prostitute, and was serving 5 to 20 years for her second conviction of drug sales, having already served 7 years on a "3 to 10" for her first offense. Because the actual length of a prisoner's sentence is ultimately determined by a state parole board, at regular hearings, board members would consider an inmate's record of behavior in prison, including participation in treatment, education, and work opportunities, and whether the prisoner had a suitable job and place to live upon parole. The indefinite sentencing model favored inmates without substance abuse or mental diagnoses who had financial resources, employment histories, and supportive, stable families. Those less fortunate served longer sentences, since the parole board would usually require them to continue their sentence until the next hearing, when perhaps somehow they could show a better parole plan. Some inmates would never be released by the board, and would eventually "max out" of prison by serving the highest number of years in their sentence.

At the time I knew Irene, nearly the entire population of the women's prison was required to complete addiction treatment in order to successfully stand before the parole board. The US War on Drugs policy instituted in the 1980s was resulting in a vast number of people with substance use problems being criminally charged and incarcerated. Our state was relatively forward-looking at the time, in that our legislature was allocating funds to treat inmates for substance abuse *during* incarceration. Alcohol and Drug Abuse Primary Treatment (ADAPT) programs at each state prison were developed and administered by a private drug treatment agency on contract to the Department of Corrections.

Our program was considered state of the art, not only as an in-prison drug treatment model, but also for specializing in women's issues. The 90-day program was closed (participants who attritioned out would not be replaced); the 32 women at the top of the ADAPT waiting list were moved into a separate dorm block where they would live and participate in treatment together. Mornings of each weekday were free for them to engage in other activities on the main compound such as a work detail or high school diploma classes. Within our program, each participant was assigned to an individual counselor for weekly sessions, and to another counselor for "small group," which was daily afternoon group therapy with seven other participants. Psychoeducational activities, lectures, and guest speakers took place mostly in "big group" with all 32 women, during the evenings and on Saturdays.

Irene had been assigned to me for her individual counselor. At her last appearance before the parole board, their verdict had been "continued for ADAPT." If she successfully finished the program, she would be paroled out of prison immediately.

Now in her 30s, Irene had grown up in an inner-city environment with her single mother who also had a substance abuse problem. Irene had worked as a prostitute and occasionally trafficked drugs for her pimp; *he* always managed to evade arrest. Irene was known for her occasional anger issues and her more-than-typical reticence to talk about her past; during all the various legal and treatment evaluations she had been through, she had been unwilling to speak about her personal history or whether there was trauma history. This was not particularly a red flag, since the typical corrections psychologist was an older white man in a suit who was likely to carry the transference identity of a prosecuting attorney or a hypocritical "john." I found Irene to be reasonable and cooperative, even likeable, and we developed a positive relationship. But even with my gentle encouragement I, too, found her to be reticent to share very much. In individual sessions, we focused on structured skill-building activities to work on relationship boundaries and relapse prevention.

Because our women's ADAPT program had no predecessor and the funding mechanism was not specific about curriculum, our contract employer gave us the freedom to design it from the ground up, and we were continually seeking to improve it. We liked to include art activities—a couple of us counselors considered ourselves artists. Although it seems incredible as I write this now, none of us had heard of the profession of art therapy. Our training and credentials were in addictions or social work. We had dim hand-me-down conceptions of psychological tasks such as family drawings, which we found to be powerful ways to jumpstart discussions in small group. At one point, knowing that some of our participants could not read or write very well, we decided to allow visual journaling as an optional alternative to our journal requirement. The results were more effective than we anticipated, and we began to actively encourage visual journaling for everyone. In groups, we sometimes made magazine collages with a pertinent theme; this seemed popular, regardless of a participant's art ability, and seemed to stimulate verbal processing. We reviewed our ideas and trial runs in our counselor bullpen and refined what seemed to be working. It was an exciting experience.

The counselors alternated working with the big group on Saturdays. One of my Saturday programs included a lecture on the developmental models of addiction and recovery in the morning, and an art-making change of pace for the afternoon. I asked each woman to make a collage using both sides of a poster board, with one side showing what it was like "before" and the other what it would be like when they "got out." I left the directions purposely somewhat vague, to allow participants to interpret them as they wished. Most women would show pictures of unhappiness or chaos on the before side; the future side was usually a ridiculously unlikely depiction of luxury. This seemed to reflect an inability to imagine a more honest, humble, in-between life—and, of course, most of the participants had never experienced one. Instead, they indulged in fantasy, choosing images of ultimate affluence (such as a beautiful woman in *haute couture* stepping from a Porsche) or exotic depictions of "serenity" (a rose-gold tropical sunset over an oceanfront property).

We counselors had reflected on this typical response to the future collage, and decided not to insist on reality. The actual future after prison for most of these women would be far from easy. Until their max date was reached, they would meet regularly with a parole officer in the community and would be required to stay sober and employed. Many would return to their children and the demands of single parenthood. They would need to set boundaries, while still wanting relationships, with partners or families still entrenched in the drug culture. Most would experience difficulty finding or keeping an adequate job with limited education, skills, and work history, and have to deal with unreliable transportation and child care; all this, while trying to maintain sobriety. We decided that we were spending plenty of time on future-serving activities like stress management, cognitive and emotional reframing, assertiveness skills, and identifying personal relapse triggers. We wanted to allow the women to play with beautiful images—to experience aesthetic pleasure and to indulge in the human need to *wish*, and symbolically and unconsciously, to portray every prisoner's desire to *escape*. Although we did not know how to articulate it, we had discovered the benefits of *art psychotherapy* via the visual journaling processed with an individual counselor, and *art as therapy* via this engagement with beautiful pictures.

At the end of one of my Saturday sessions, all participants except Irene had completed their two-sided collages and shared them willingly. As usual, there was a lot of luxury depicted in the "after" side, and a range of personal honesty in the "before" sides; some focused on the drugs or violence in their environments, others portrayed their own personal failures or traumatic experiences. Irene showed me that she had cut out a few images, but said that she would not share until she had completed the collage. She requested permission to ask the dorm correctional officer to add the poster board and images to her property list, so she could take them back to her cell until she was finished. This procedure was accomplished, and I soon forgot that she had not completed the project.

At the end of the 90-day treatment cycle, those who had completed the program (it was possible to opt out or be dismissed) took part in a graduation ceremony. We collaborated to put on a special program that varied for each group: we wanted to honor them as a unique cohort and as individuals, and not to just pass out certificates of completion. Although I suspected that Irene had not been totally forthcoming about her past, I believed that she had really invested in working on her addiction; I thought she should be proud, and said so during the ceremony.

It was after I spoke that I finally recalled Irene's struggle to complete her collage poster. Then, after the ceremony, she brought it to my office and said she wanted me to have it. She shrugged as she explained that she hadn't really followed directions or used both sides, and that she just hadn't wanted to turn it in before. She had already taken care of the paperwork to release the poster for my use. She didn't stay in the office long enough for me to read the rather extensive captions next to the images; instead, she smiled and thanked me for being her counselor. Then she promptly joined the rest of the women, who were busy saying their goodbyes as they packed, some to move back onto the main compound and others, including Irene, to parole out to a relative waiting at the gate. The dorm would quickly be emptied to make way for the next group of participants from the ADAPT waiting list.

Although this happened over 25 years ago and I have moved jobs and homes several times since, I still have Irene's collage. After she had left my office, I read the captions, and gasped; the images had not been alarming at first glance, but they became chillingly evocative in conjunction with the material revealed in her labels and typed captions. Overtly, there was not a bit of Irene's personal story or drawing on the poster, yet the piece powerfully represented her personal effort to achieve verbal articulation and intellectualization of her experience of being raped. She had painstakingly typed labels from another source and paired them with her own evocative choice of images, which, as I knew from being in the room that Saturday, had taken her 90 minutes to choose. It seemed the directive prompt and images had inspired for her a safe way to communicate to me the fact of her experience, even if I would never know if the rape was a singular event or many, had occurred during her childhood, in her life on the street, or more recently, in the prison.

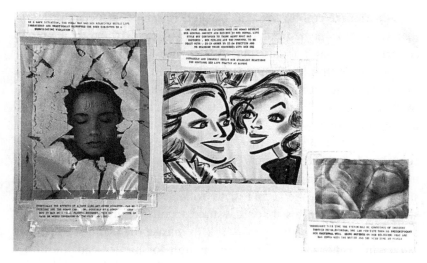

Figure P.1: Irene's collage. Irene used colored pencils to write words directly on the first image: on the woman's forehead, "DREAM," and on the shattered material surrounding her face, "ENORMOUS AGITATION," "SHOCK," "CRY + HYSTERIA," and "ANXIETY" (see color plate)

I later pieced together her method for completing the collage by talking with correctional staff. Irene used to spend some of her free time at the small prison library, and had been observed reading a psychology textbook and using the old standard typewriter there to take notes. Later, in the office of the dorm correctional officer, she borrowed scissors and tape to trim and adhere the papers and images to her poster. The material she typed is reproduced below. I have assumed that the errors, abridgement, and bolding are hers, not the unknown textbook author's. It should be noted that typewriters had no simple "bold" function. To bold something required that the typist backspace to the correct position and strike each letter key again, usually multiple times, to achieve a dark effect. This would contribute to a kinesthetic, perhaps therapeutic, feeling of emphasis. Irene also did not bother with switching from upper to lower case, and the all-caps presentation denotes a sense of forcefulness.

> (Above picture on left) IN A RAPE SITUATION, THE WOMAN HAS HAD HER RELATIVELY SECURE LIFE THREATENED AND **DRASTICALLY DISRUPTED** SHE BEEN SUBJECTED TO A **HUNMILIATING VIOLATION**
>
> (Below picture on left) EVENTUALLY THE EFFECTS OF A RAPE LIKE ANY OTHER DISASTER, CAN BE OVERCOME AND THE WOMAN CAN GO ON, POSSIBLY AS A STRONGER PERSON BUT IT MAY BE A LONG, PAINFUL RECOVERY. THIS MAY BE A MATTER OF DAYS OR WEEKS DEPENDING ON THE VICT AND CIRCUMSTANCES
>
> (Middle picture) THE FIRT PHASE IS FINISHED WHEN THE WOMAN RESOLVE HER GENERAL ANXIETY AND RETURNS TO HER NORMAL LIFE STYLE BUT CONTINUES TO THINK ABOUT WHAT HAS HAPPENED, HER FEELING ARE TOO POWERFUL TO BE DEALT WITH. SO IN ORDER TO GO ON FUNCTION AND TO REASSURE THOSE CONCERNED WITH HER SHE OUTWARDLY AND INWARDLY DENIES HER STRONGEST REACTIONS SHE CONTINUE HER LIFE EXACTLY AS BEFORE
>
> (Picture on right) THROUGHOUT THIS TIME THE VICTIM MAY BE CONSCIOUS OF INCIDENT THROUGH DREAM, DAYDREAM, SHE CAN PERCEIVE THEM AS **INSIGNIFICANT** HER **EMOTIONAL WELL BEING DEPENDS** ON HER BELIEVING THAT SHE HAS COPED WITH THE MATTER AND SHE NEED TIME TO ADJUST

I was certainly not new to the dynamic wherein a client who is due to terminate suddenly "remembers" some major issue that needs attention, but Irene had waited until she had totally completed the program and was beyond my therapeutic reach before she shared her secret! I felt simultaneously anguished, frustrated, thrilled, and honored. Over the ensuing years, the collage stayed in my office and prompted my thoughts about the power of images and art making to communicate in therapy.

Irene's collage was to have another important role to play in my life. It was still lying on a work table in my office a short time after Irene paroled out, when one of our guest speakers stopped by to say hi after her presentation. Her name was Marilynn Ault, and I knew her only as the director of the city's domestic violence agency. She had a warm and direct style with the women, and we appreciated her volunteering to talk with them about relationship abuse.

Marilynn glanced at the collage and said, "Oh! You're doing art therapy!" I chuckled; since I didn't realize that "art therapy" was an actual approach or field, I thought she was being facetious. She sensed my ignorance and added, "It's a true profession; in fact, my husband founded a master's degree program here in Kansas at Emporia State, about 20 years ago." I was stunned. This meant that at the very time I had been working on my undergraduate degree, as I dreamed and longed for some special training or job that would combine psychology and art, unbeknownst to me or my undergrad faculty advisor, art therapy pioneer Robert Ault was establishing one of the first master's in art therapy at a university not 60 miles from mine. (This kind of ignorance could only have happened prior to the internet!)

I had chosen my undergraduate university because students were allowed to design their own bachelor's degrees. I had put together a BA in humanities with coursework in art, literature, psychology, and philosophy, and titled my senior comprehensive "The Examined Life: Understandings of Existence in Literature and Philosophy"—which is actually emblazoned on my transcript as the degree title. It was a glorious experience, but prepared me for absolutely no career that I could discover, and after several years working as a bartender, I found my footing again and decided to become an addictions counselor. I went back to college, earned an academic certificate in addictions counseling, and began work in that field. At the time, when master's degrees in addictions counseling had not yet been established, the acquisition of a master's in social work was *de rigueur* for career advancement. I had been pondering this rather glumly for a few years. Now Marilynn was suggesting I visit her husband at his studio private practice and chat about the master's degree in art therapy! I certainly needed no further encouragement, but I remember her adding, "He's really a nice man."

Bob Ault was indeed one of the kindest people I have ever known. We spent many hours together in the later years of his life, painting and sharing ideas about the provision and profession of art therapy. Throughout his supervision of me as a student intern, then as my ATR (Registered Art Therapist) credentialing supervisor, and later as a mentor for my own studio model private practice and teaching at the program he founded, Bob was a support and an inspiration. His influence remains at the heart of my delight in the art and the stories.

Introduction

Similarities of the professions and scope of this book

The profession of addiction counseling is similar to that of art therapy in several ways. Although it has existed in some form or another for years, addiction counseling is relatively new as a full profession in its own right. There are a limited number of graduate-level training programs specifically in the field, and although national credentials are strong, the presence or rigor of state government credentialing is wide-ranging. The profession must compete with more well-established ones for parity in funding, licensure, and employment. At the local level, qualified practitioners may struggle to be heard as experts in their own field when they are on the same treatment team with other types of professionals.

Addiction-specific educational requirements within degrees in related fields, such as social work, psychology, and even clinical counseling and medicine, are still minimal, where they exist, except in degree specializations. Perhaps because of this, some of these professionals assume that there is not much to know, or that expertise in their own profession trumps the need for specific knowledge of addiction. It is difficult to convince those with such assumptions that there is indeed much to know. The acquisition of at least a modicum of this specialized knowledge is important, not just for the treatment of people whose presenting problem is substance abuse, but also to inform understandings of a preponderance of all mental health clients.

So, while this book was written in particular because a gap was perceived in the art therapy literature, particularly with regard to textbooks, readers should not expect to receive adequate knowledge of addictions to consider themselves specialists by reading this book. Art therapists working in addictions treatment who do not otherwise have addictions training are encouraged to pursue continuing education, take specialty college classes, and read. Good information is readily available—a starting list of resources is provided in Appendix B. For those without personal experience of addiction and recovery, attending open meetings of Alcoholics Anonymous® (AA) or Narcotics Anonymous® (NA) provides insight into the experience of addiction and recovery.

Along the same lines, those who are not art therapists are advised that reading this book is not a substitute for training as a professional art therapist, which requires a master's degree in art therapy and subsequent supervised experience in the provision of art therapy for credentialing. If other mental health professionals choose to employ therapeutic art activities, it is highly recommended that they first do the activity themselves, and try to imagine the range of responses that their clients might have. Facilitators are often surprised at how quickly and deeply the art can access emotions or buried trauma. When this occurs unexpectedly, especially in a group setting where the safety of multiple clients is at stake, the facilitator must be prepared to respond appropriately. Those not possessing the appropriate credential must also take care not to state that they are art therapists or providing art therapy, or to analyze or interpret clients' art. It should be noted that the latter is something that trained art therapists themselves do only in certain situations, always with appropriate reservations, and usually by engaging the client in a nonleading manner.

Art therapy and addictions also have in common a great potential for expansion of research and support of best practices by the burgeoning field of neuroscience. This topic is one that deserves considerable attention, but can be addressed only briefly in this book, where it is seen as one way among others to conceptualize the disease of addiction and to inform art therapy approaches to treatment.

I urge readers to realize how vastly heterogeneous the substance abuse treatment (SAT) population is. People of all ages, ethnicities, cultures, socioeconomic standings, educational levels, abilities, gender identities, and sexual orientations present with substance use problems. It is not within the scope of this book to provide training for each of these aspects of diversity and their derivatives, although vignettes featuring people from nondominant cultures are given throughout the book, and a brief focus on the subpopulation of adolescents is provided in Chapter 8. Failure of this book to mention or cover any specific special population or need is not meant to insinuate that it is not important or does not have special considerations within these fields, or that there is a dearth of literature and resources concerning special groups.

Case material and illustrations

The material used in the vignettes and case examples is taken from actual cases, but pseudonyms are used and other particulars may have been changed to further protect confidentiality. All those whose case material or art was used in this book provided informed consent. A few of the client artworks were recreated due to the original photographic records being of poor quality. A few of the other illustrations were made by students or others not participating in art therapy; they are also reproduced with permission of the artist.

A note on use of terms and acronyms

Accepted terminology in the field of addiction has changed over the years. All mental health professionals are now trained in the importance of using person-first language when referring to those with disabilities or diagnoses. In preparing this book, however, I found the flow of writing hampered by continually having to refer to the population as *people who misuse alcohol or other drugs*. Acceptable terms for people accessing treatment like *service users* also become awkward when used repetitively. Therefore, I have tried to vary terms, sometimes using *client*, which is still common where I live; *patient* for those in inpatient settings; *participant* for those in groups; or simply *people*. I have also chosen to make use of certain established acronyms for the sake of brevity, without spelling out their meaning after the first use: PWAI for *people with addiction issues* (a broader category than *clients* in that it includes those who have not accessed treatment), SUD for *substance use disorders*, and SAT for *substance abuse treatment* (see the List of Acronyms).

The commonly heard phrase *alcohol and drugs* implies that alcohol is different and somehow safer or better than other psychoactive drugs; however, alcohol operates on the brain like any other addictive drug. A push to use the term *alcohol and other drugs* (AOD) has been successful in the profession, if not in the speech of the public. In addition to using this acronym in the text, I use the word *drug* to refer to any psychoactive drug that may be abused, including alcohol and prescription varieties.

The *Diagnostic and Statistical Manual of Mental Disorders, 5th Edition* (DSM-5) diagnostic title *alcohol use disorder* is the preferred replacement for the term *alcoholism*. When speaking about substance addiction generally or with regard to research, *addiction* is still appropriate. An individual, if so diagnosed, may be described as having a SUD, or as having the particular DSM diagnosis (which is named for the drug being abused, e.g., methamphetamine use disorder). In the battle against stigma, it has been recommended that professionals in the field do not use the terms *addict* or *alcoholic* during the provision of treatment, even when speaking generically in psychoeducational sessions. In some self-help groups, participants are encouraged to use the term *alcoholic* or *addict* when introducing themselves, arguably for good reasons, but the ultimate decision is up to the individual.

Whereas *clean and sober* was once the term of choice for abstinence from both drugs and alcohol, the term *sober* is now used more broadly to encompass abstinence from AOD. People who are coming from certain self-help and treatment programs may refer to themselves in sobriety as a *recovering* person, alcoholic, or addict, which alludes to the continual need for abstinence; *recovered* is thought wrongly to insinuate having achieved a cure that allows a return to normal substance use. Other people with long-term abstinence may choose to refer to themselves as *recovered*, as *former* addicts, or as being in recovery or working a program of recovery; it is best left to the individual to provide self-definition, if any is to be given.

Finally, although counselors are the professionals who most often work with this population, in this book the term *therapist* is used broadly to refer to both art therapists and substance abuse professionals.

List of acronyms

The following acronyms may be encountered in the text and citations without being spelled out first:

AA Alcoholics Anonymous®
ADHD Attention deficit hyperactivity disorder

AOD Alcohol and/or other drugs

ATCB Art Therapy Credentials Board, credentialing body for professional art therapists

CDC US Centers for Disease Control and Prevention

CSAT, SAMHSA Center for Substance Abuse Treatment, a division of the Substance Abuse and Mental Health Services Administration of the US government; it facilitates delivery of services and grants in prevention and treatment programs, and compiles educational materials for professionals and the public

DSM-5 The current 5th edition of the *Diagnostic Statistical Manual of Mental Disorders*, the diagnostic manual of the American Psychiatric Association

ETC Expressive Therapies Continuum, a developmental model for arts therapies

GHB Gamma-hydroxybutyrate, a sedative sometimes used to facilitate sexual assault

HIV, AIDS Human immunodeficiency virus, acquired immune deficiency syndrome

K-F-D Kinetic Family Drawing, originally a psychological projective assessment, now sometimes used therapeutically or informally

K-H-T-P Kinetic House-Tree-Person drawing, originally a psychological projective assessment, now sometimes used therapeutically or informally

LGBTQ Lesbian, gay, bisexual, transsexual, queer (or questioning)

LSD Lysergic acid diethylamide, a laboratory-produced psychedelic drug of abuse

MDMA 3,4-Methylenedioxymethamphetamine, also known as ecstasy, a hallucinogenic drug of abuse

NA Narcotics Anonymous®

NAADAC Originally an acronym for the National Association of Alcohol and Drug Abuse Counselors, but having expanded to include gambling and other types of addictions, it is now referred to as NAADAC, the Association for Addiction Professionals

NCADD National Council on Alcoholism and Drug Dependence, a powerful non-governmental advocacy organization with regional offices that educates the public and professionals, fights stigma, lobbies for treatment legislation, and helps individuals find appropriate services through national and regional offices

NIDA, NIAAA, NIH National Institute on Drug Abuse, and National Institute on Alcohol Abuse and Alcoholism, of the US National Institutes of Health (NIH), research institutes and providers of extensive and reliable information about substances of abuse and addiction to inform best practices in policy, education, prevention, and treatment

PTSD Post-traumatic stress disorder

PWAI People (or person) with addiction issues

SAT Substance abuse treatment

SSRI Selective serotonin reuptake inhibitors, a class of prescription antidepressants

SUD Substance use disorders

THC Delta-9-tetrahydrocannabinol, the primary psychoactive component of marijuana

UK United Kingdom

US United States

1
Findings in the Art Therapy Literature

The first published article referencing the use of art therapy to treat substance abuse appears to have been a 1953 contribution to *Psychiatry* by art therapy pioneer Elinor Ulman, which described her work at the Alcoholic Rehabilitation Program of the District of Colombia. My search has turned up approximately 80 sources since that time. Other reviewers of the literature, including Moore (1983) and Mahony and Waller (1992), commented on the lack of published material on this population, especially of research. This still may be said, although perhaps the lack should not be very surprising since the specialty field is so small, and the substance abuse treatment (SAT) population is protected, at least at many settings in the United States, from being used as research participants. Much of the literature in the US has focused on spirituality or the Twelve Steps. More recent additions have addressed the incorporation of art therapy into newer SAT approaches such as Motivational Interviewing (MI) and the Transtheoretical Model (TTM) or Stages of Change (SOC), or explored art therapy applications such as the Expressive Therapies Continuum (ETC) or the Bird's Nest Drawing (BND).

This chapter provides a selective look at key points in the literature. As I researched and read, I was continually impressed with the potential helpfulness of all, even the oldest, material. Except where other citations are needed to provide background, citations found in this chapter represent readings in which both art therapy and the substance abuse population are referenced predominantly. Professional art therapists wrote almost all of this material. Subsequent chapters in this book will revisit some of these sources as well as referencing additional ones.

Psychodynamically informed approaches

In the earlier years of the art therapy profession in the US, and still in the United Kingdom (Woods and Springham 2011), art therapists have favored psychodynamic approaches. This theoretical orientation is not supported in the general practice of SAT in the US, but every approach has the potential to broaden understanding. The roots of art therapy run deep in psychoanalytic theory, and psychodynamic concepts underlie cognitive, humanistic, and other dominant approaches to SAT. For example, the topic of denial and other ego defenses is standard in SAT psychoeducational groups.

In a psychodynamic model, substance abuse may be interpreted as a narcissistic defense which may involve oral fixation, and which may be resolved by working through resistance and transference and gaining insight. Albert-Puleo (1980) described the addict's retreat into a drug-induced state as a variation of the narcissistic defense. This type of defense is first established in infancy or early childhood, when the expression of normal hostile feelings toward the love object is avoided by withdrawal and turning those feelings inward. A person whose infancy needs were not met appropriately may develop an oral fixation and continue to use immature defenses or behaviors, including substance abuse, in a search for comfort. Rubin (2005) wrote that those with addiction issues might find nonverbal modes of expression congenial, due to the origin of unresolved issues in early life when language was not well developed. Painting or drawing may replace or enhance the traditional psychoanalyst's tools of dream work and free association. The presence of the art product modifies transference, usually in a positive way (Rubin 2011).

Springham (1999) discussed the development of the false self within this population. This persona becomes whatever the love object or environmental pressures demand, and in the process overrides the true self that is capable of feeling and communicating honestly. Springham observed the operation of this dynamic when clients "say all the right things to their therapist with considerable accuracy, but make no development emotionally" (1999, p.9). In other words, the false self continues to operate in order to reduce the likelihood of a disagreeable relationship with the current object or authority figure. Art therapy can offer a way to reduce the split of the false and true selves by allowing clients to express themselves more honestly through the art and to experience and accept ambivalence in self-identity.

Springham (1999) worked in a relatively nondirective manner with regard to art making in groups. Progress was often revealed during the group verbal processing of the individuals' art products. When working individually with substance abusers, Albert-Puleo (1980) also worked nondirectively. She would provide any instruction needed for use of the art materials, then sit behind and outside the patient's vision, while the patient sat facing an easel with a spot-lit blank canvas and painted whatever came to mind. The art itself, in addition to being a tool for communication, was a receptacle for unacceptable client feelings: impulses could be discharged into the art product, rather than being repressed or avoided by drug abuse. The art therapist played a supportive rather than directive role as the client emerged from the narcissistic reverie achieved in the painting process. In group settings, Albert-Puleo and Osha (1976–77) viewed the art therapist's role as modeling communication, making interpretive responses, and pointing out overlooked symbolism. Encouraging client interpretations facilitated the development of insight.

Having been inspired by Kohut's theories of narcissism, Lachman-Chapin (1979) described the power of art in working individually with this population. In particular, she identified the grandiosity that is often cited as characteristic of substance abusers—the inflated sense of self that seeks to be seen and hailed by all others. Lachman-Chapin wrote that the traditional neutral role of a psychotherapist, designed to encourage the transference, was not well suited or necessary to art therapy. Instead, she promoted a mirroring transference approach, which addresses the grandiose nature and gradually modifies it. In her own practice, she employed mirroring in two ways: by observing and admiring as the client created self-objects in their art, and by creating art alongside the client in a way that mirrored their work. Either approach provided the client with the gift of having their narcissistic needs understood and met, thus paving the way for the development of more mature functioning. This article provides an excellent example of how earlier work from our literature is still of value; anyone familiar with the current trends focusing on reparative attachment would see equivalences in Lachman-Chapin's process.

Kaufman (1981) noted how art products reflect patients' progress through SAT. She discussed a successful case whose initial images reflected a paranoid projection: the client defended against his inner rage by depicting a hostile world. His art evolved to include images that acknowledged his anger and depicted humans rather than abstractions. In contrast, another client never progressed beyond making drawings that reflected rigid defenses, such as masks, walls, and prison-like structures. Kaufman believed that art therapy was successful for the former client due to his ability to feel safe with the therapist and therapy group. Like Lachman-Chapin, Kaufman's style reflected an integration of psychodynamic theory with a more humanistic style presence.

Erdmann (1972) described an unmotivated client who was allowed to bring painting materials into his room in an inpatient alcoholism treatment setting. The patient worked in a self-directed manner and developed a symbolic, Dali-esque style that he became eager to interpret in individual sessions with Erdmann. Symbol interpretation and the ensuing facilitation of insight are basic to psychodynamic art therapy approaches, yet the art making also tends to balance the therapeutic relationship, making the art therapist's role less aloof than in some traditional psychoanalytic models. This patient's art production energized his treatment process; he gained insight as a partner in symbol exploration with the therapist.

Luzzatto (1987) devised a directive called the Self Image to study self–object relations in a SAT population ($n=50$) and a control group of nurses. Participants chose a shape to depict themselves, drew its outline, and then filled the inner and outer worlds appropriately. Four types emerged from her analysis: the vulnerable self, the objectless self, the divided (split) self, and the integrated self. Only 10 percent of the treatment population drawings were evaluated as integrated, compared to 80 percent of the control group drawings. Luzzatto suggested that visual treatment modalities could help these patients better understand their barriers against the world, splitting, or internalized "bad self." In her 1989 description of two case studies, Luzzatto interpreted imagery in terms of *withdrawal* and *clinging*, two behaviors identified as early responses to an unsatisfactory object relationship, which may also underlie addictive behavior in adulthood (again, these notions are addressed in modern attachment theory and research).

Incorporating art therapy into traditional substance abuse treatment

Generally and anecdotally, the art therapy literature describes integration of art therapy approaches into SAT as successful, although perhaps not always in a manner desired by the art therapist. Allen (1985) reported plainly on the limitations that are often placed on art therapy in an alcoholism treatment program. As a staff member required to serve on a rotation of psychoeducational lectures, Allen created a slide presentation of fine art that addressed the universal themes of human existence. During her presentation, clients were encouraged to verbally project feelings and discuss the work. They learned that art was part of life, that it could be used to integrate internal and external reality, and to relieve feelings and reduce isolation. Allen also provided a hands-on art therapy group with goals to reduce resistance to treatment and enlarge clients' sense of perspective. In using themes such as how spouses were affected by the client's addiction or envisioning a higher power, she was both directive and supportive. Although the lecture rotation and theme-based approaches were not those she personally favored as an art therapist, she was committed to work within the program structure. She realized that to do otherwise would be to enable splitting and confusion in the clients, perhaps causing them to reject her message about the importance of art altogether.

Several other art therapists have written about incorporating art therapy into existing programs. Mahony (1999) explored the use of art activities and art therapy in 16 SAT programs in the UK. Her qualitative review identified three major themes or uses for the art: educative (learn to think creatively, leisure interests); healing (expressing feelings, catharsis); and psychotherapeutic (enabling communication and further interventions in therapy). Dickson (2007) used client questionnaires to evaluate the addition of art therapy to a residential drug treatment program; two-thirds of respondents found both art and verbal aspects of treatment to be valuable. She observed that clients appeared to better develop reflective functioning through the art experiences. Wadeson (2000, 2010) described working on issues of substance abuse in a variety of settings where clients had presented with comorbid conditions. She reported on the successful use of clay with inpatient clients whose drawing style tended to be over-controlled, which reflected their desire to "give the right answer" (2000, p.206). Smashing and reforming the clay was more permissible than making mistakes in a drawing, and enabled discussion of metaphors such as loss of control and starting over. I have previously (2006) described a curriculum of art therapy in SAT programming for women with comorbid issues including borderline personality, eating disorder, drug-assisted date rape, childhood sexual trauma, and domestic abuse. Art therapy enabled reduction of shame and a clearer understanding of personal life patterns, and promoted other goals such as learning assertiveness skills, connecting with other women, and appropriately expressing emotions.

Motivational Interviewing and the Stages of Change

The Transtheoretical Model (TTM) (Prochaska, DiClemente, and Norcross 1992), which includes and is also informally referred to as the Stages of Change (SOC), and Motivational Interviewing (MI), (Miller and Rollnick 2013, first published 1991) are theoretical and practical treatment models that were developed independently and have been refined, applied, and researched for decades. Their principles are congruent and the two are frequently mentioned together; they find great support in current SAT practice. Rather than espousing a confrontational style to break denial, counselors work in a cooperative, compassionate manner to embody the so-called spirit of MI and enable clients' innate motivation to change.

Several art therapists have designed protocols to fit MI/SOC frameworks. Art therapist Horay (2006) described working with a client using an MI/SOC approach and interventions such as a pro/con collage, hypothetical greeting cards, and check-in drawings to explore the client's ambivalence and motivation, promote self-efficacy, and encourage movement away from rigid thinking and expectations. Holt and Kaiser (2009) devised a protocol of five art therapy directives called the First Step Series that focuses on the early SOC using MI tactics such as targeting denial, normalizing ambivalence, and supporting internal desire to change. Their crisis directive requires clients to depict the crisis or event that brought them to treatment. Their recovery bridge directive identifies the bridge as a metaphor for the passage to recovery. The protocol was completed by a cost–benefits collage, a two-drawing task to *depict yourself a year from now, both if change is made and if it is not*, and a barriers-to-recovery drawing.

Diehls (2008) used the Stages of Change Readiness and Treatment Eagerness Scale (SOCRATES) to assess movement toward change in 12 participants in art therapy during SAT. Her protocol featured the incident drawing (Cox and Price 1990), the pro/con collage

(Horay 2006), the bridge drawing (Hays and Lyons 1981), and a self-esteem collage (*assemble images representing your strengths*), which were chosen to suggest sequential movement through the SOC. Diehls found statistically significant improvement of SOCRATES scores within and between SOC. Palmer (2014) discussed art therapy applications focusing on three aspects of MI: resistance, ambivalence, and readiness. She found that therapist-facilitated exploration of themed directives, such as to depict the balancing act involved in making a choice, helped clients identify internal struggles and secondary gains as issues underlying ambivalence toward treatment.

Crowe and Parmenter (2012) reviewed the literature on creative approaches to MI and identified specific expressive arts (visual art, writing, movement, and drama) techniques and directives, including some of those mentioned above, that apply to the four key principles of MI: expressing empathy, developing discrepancy, rolling with resistance, and supporting self-efficacy.

Other addiction approaches and settings

Short-term hospital-based inpatient settings

These settings generally feature patients with comorbid conditions who are in crisis. Matto (2002) cited the usefulness of art therapy in this setting to aid in assessment, facilitate therapeutic change, and track and document patient progress. Her article included a discussion of appropriate theoretical orientations, guidelines for verbal processing, and ideas for directives.

Detoxification approach

Feen-Calligan (2007) described an approach for incorporating art therapy to support the three goals of a detoxification program: by assisting identification of issues in medical withdrawal via art assessment; by supporting humane and dignified withdrawal by introducing aesthetic experiences in healing relationships; and by preparing clients for ongoing treatment by identifying issues such as barriers to recovery. Tasks such as creative journaling allowed clients to continue to benefit after detoxification as they awaited entry into a treatment program.

Harm reduction approach

This pragmatic approach is used to reduce the negative consequences of drug abuse without insisting on abstinence or even changing the level of use. For example, it may involve the use of clean needles for injection drug users to reduce the risk of disease, or installing devices in vehicles that prevent driving when one has been drinking. Wise (2009) described an open art studio in an inner-city harm reduction center whose primary goal was to reduce the spread of HIV in substance users. Fresh materials for drawing, painting, and collage were provided for specific periods of time, and participation was open to studio regulars as well as drop-ins who were there for the other services. The art studio became a place where participants could know and share more about themselves than just their problems with substance use, homelessness, or HIV. Humor and empathy were identified as natural healing outcomes.

Solution-focused therapy

This treatment approach builds on learning from past successes and identifying and using strengths to develop approaches to problems. Matto, Corcoran, and Fassler (2003) discussed the compatibility of this approach with art therapy in SAT, and provided ideas for directives that correlate to solution-focused techniques, as well as lists of process-guiding questions for verbal exploration.

Family therapy

Family therapy may be recommended as an adjunct to a client's SAT, or may be sought by others in the family. Perkoulidis (2009) provided suggestions for creating a multifamily group art-therapy program to address the needs of families with substance-using adolescents. Benefits include bonding via family-friendly activities, the shame-reducing structure of peer support for both/all generations of family members, and reduction of the stigma attached to attendance at traditional drug treatment programs. Ranganathan and Malick (2013) described a one-month inpatient treatment program in India that is provided to families of patients. One or more family members attend two-weekly arts-based therapy groups with the patient. Use of story, music, and drama is supported in the Indian culture and helped the families internalize information and insights; the authors provided specific suggestions for making cultural adaptations for Western art therapists working with this population. McClean (1999) described how art psychotherapy helped facilitate the working-through of dependency conflicts in a child living at a long-term residential program with her mother who was undergoing SAT. McClean found that the defense mechanisms of the children at the setting often mirrored those of their substance-abusing parents.

Holistic approaches

The holistic model in SAT includes programming or services such as meditation or mindfulness interventions, spiritual or religious opportunities, acupuncture, yoga, tai chi, cultural appreciation, and expressive arts. The value of art therapy within this approach lies in its ability to enhance emotional regulation and self-expression, promote self-esteem, and allow deep healing through the creative process. Those writing about addiction treatment in other professions from social work to nursing have recognized the value of art therapy within a holistic model (Adedoyin *et al.* 2014; Aletraris *et al.* 2014; Breslin, Reed, and Malone 2003).

Expressive and creative arts therapies

Several authors have explored the range of expressive arts therapies as beneficial to the treatment of substance abuse. Adelman and Castricone (1986) cited the overdeveloped defense mechanisms found in the addiction population as a reason to add expressive therapies to the traditional verbal counseling approach. They described an expressive arts model that integrated psychodrama, art therapy, and music therapy in group work to aid substance abuse clients in self-expression, self-discovery, and the development of empathy for others. Haluzan (2012) wrote that art and music-based activities improve overall functioning by stimulating the sensory system and enabling relaxed communication. Harms (1973) wrote that art activity satisfies innate needs for play and action, and presented a case where ultimately the client became so involved in art making that his drug dependence was seen as interfering with the creative impulse. Both Harms and Head (1975) have written of the stimulant effect of art making on those who have been addicted to pharmacological depressants, or who are experiencing depression in sobriety.

Scott and Ross (2006) identified eight processes essential to the provision of art therapy, including catharsis, sublimation, and integration. They described the integration of a range of expressive techniques and directives into treatment for trauma and addictions. Biley (2006) identified a distinctive benefit of incorporating expressive arts in SAT. He stated that professional counselors who are not demographically or experientially similar to their substance-abusing clients tend to have negative attitudes toward those clients. However, counselors' understanding of their clients' experience is improved by witnessing the expressive presentations that convey the addict experience in a stark and vivid manner.

Two edited books (Brooke 2009; Waller and Mahony 1999) explore expressive arts approaches to SAT. These appear to be the only published books containing information about professional art therapy approaches in SAT prior to this one, although many books and workbooks have been written about creativity and recovery. These two edited books feature chapters on various creative arts therapies including music, dance/movement, poetry, and drama.

Assessment
Assessment-related research
Art therapists have researched and written about the use of art tasks as diagnostic or prognostic tools within the addiction population. Francis, Kaiser, and Deaver (2003) administered a demographic profile, a relationship questionnaire, and the Bird's Nest Drawing (BND) and story (an assessment task devised to gauge attachment security; see Kaiser 1996) to a group of patients with diagnosed substance use disorders (SUD) and to a control group with no known history of substance abuse. Those with SUD were more likely to have insecure attachment; content analysis found themes of aggression and anger combined with those of family and food in the stories provided by those in the substance abuse group. Francis *et al.* recommended a treatment emphasis on skills for developing stable relationships to support recovery.

Rockwell and Dunham (2006) researched the utility of the Formal Elements Art Therapy Scale (FEATS) (Gantt and Tabone 1998;

Gantt 2001) to assess SUD. Two otherwise-matched groups, one of which was composed of those diagnosed with SUD, were administered the Person Picking an Apple from a Tree (PPAT) drawing, which was scored using the FEATS. The groups were distinguished with 85 percent accuracy. Statistical analysis indicated that three of the 12 FEATS scales accurately predicted SUD: Realism (SUD drawings featured fewer details); Developmental (SUD drawings were more two-dimensional); and Person (SUD drawings tended to feature stick figures rather than dimensional people).

Recognizing the impact of parental alcoholism on children, Holt and Kaiser (2001) explored use of the Kinetic Family Drawing (K-F-D) by administering it to two groups of children (total $n=34$), one with parents identified with alcoholism and the other with no known parental alcoholism. Two of the six items on their evaluation scale reached significance for children of alcoholics: depiction of isolation of self and depiction of isolation of other family members.

Dickman, Dunn, and Wolf (1996) explored the usefulness of artwork made in treatment for predicting post-treatment relapse. Their five-year retrospective study identified three potential markers for relapse: depiction of drugs or drug paraphernalia; lack of an articulated figure; and use of an abstract or geometric drawing style on at least two-thirds of the picture.

Commonly occurring symbols and themes

Many authors have written about symbolic motifs, content, or style that appear to be characteristic of the drawings of substance abuse clients. Water has been cited frequently as a common element in drawings. Albert-Puleo and Osha (1976–77) reported images of streams, wells, seascapes, and boats on water among their clientele with alcoholism; they identified one meaning as the longing for regressive security (a return to the womb), which may be simultaneously longed for, denied, and resented. This dynamic is also reflected in alcoholic behavior toward the bottle. Thus, water drawings may reflect dependency needs and self-destructive or ambivalent fantasies. In her work with men with alcoholism, Devine (1970) found that boats, water, and crosses were frequently depicted in nondirective art tasks, but that depiction of human figures was avoided. As treatment progressed, her clients' art became looser and less controlled, suggesting reduced guardedness and a greater comfort level with feelings. In a professional presentation in 1979, Gantt and Howie observed that drawings by those with alcoholism often focused on themes of ambivalence, jobs, depression, denial, grief, and symbols such as boats and water (cited in Moore 1983). Wadeson (2010) listed clouds, ambivalence, loss, the passage of time, and incidents of substance use as frequently depicted content in drawings by clients in an outpatient drug treatment center.

In examining 100 drawings of 26 patients who were chronic users of illicit drugs, Naitove (1976) identified 20 recurrent symbols or motifs. The most frequently depicted were geometric patterns, blood, eyes, and pills. She found that frank discussion of symbolic content of their art helped patients derive insight and interact in group art therapy on a more meaningful level.

Spring (1985) noted characteristic symbols in drawings of women in SAT who had been sexually abused. Wedge shapes and eyes, which she had identified as markers of sexual abuse in her earlier work with trauma survivors, were present, but dulled. Additionally, she found a predominance of red flowers, as well as faces, people, and water, in the early stages of drug treatment. These waned over time, and as they moved into recovery, this population often integrated the original wedge and eye forms into positive and skillful artwork.

Springham (1992) reported on the commonplace production of images that reflected a yearning for "the peace of pre-ambivalence" (p.9), such as images identified by clients as the light at the end of the tunnel, the bright future, or the paradise by the sea. In a later manuscript (1999), Springham refined the concept of "paradise pictures" (p.153), and gave examples such as a pastoral landscape of the client enjoying nature with his dog or a tropical island. He found such drawings to be indicative of narcissistic processes—the overly idealized object and the issues of entitlement—and made a distinction between these and the picturesque art products described in other art therapy literature that have a more integrated or communicative property.

Ault (ca. 1976) wrote of people with substance use issues within the hippie subculture, and speculated that a sensation-seeking motivation for drug use was reflected in characteristics of the art. He identified these common features as fluidity of line, the incorporation of graffiti-style words or poetry into a design, use of nonharmonious color combinations and other optical effects that create a sense of movement, and subject matter chosen for shock value. Teasdale (1993) found that the quality of work by clients who had abused hard drugs (sic) tended to be more openly excessive, "pouring out feelings and ideas" (p.17), which readily provided fodder for further work, while the imagery of alcoholics was usually more restrained and introverted.

Hanes (2007) explored self-portraits spontaneously produced by clients in SAT and observed that they may signify a readiness or need to come "face to face" with their addiction. The drawings he observed provided an accurate self-image or fitting symbolism; he believed the drawings assisted the clients in overcoming denial. Kaufman (1981) wrote about the use of drawings to generate rapid assessment impressions, such as identifying patients who were at risk for becoming violent, getting high, or leaving treatment.

Metaphorical or projective directives

Several metaphorical drawing tasks have been described as useful for informal assessment or as therapeutic interventions with the substance abuse population. These include bridge drawing (Hays and Lyons 1981), road drawing (Hanes 1995), the amusement park technique (Hrenko and Willis 1996), Bird's Nest Drawing (BND) (Kaiser 1996), and Draw a Person in the Rain (DAPR) (Willis, Joy, and Kaiser 2010). Some of these are examined further in Chapter 4.

Group work

Springham (1998) provided a helpful look at therapy group characteristics and dynamics within the SAT population, and the effect of art therapy on group processes. Although he explored these issues from a psychodynamic perspective, his portrait accurately depicts the pitfalls likely to befall the therapist, no matter which orientation is preferred. (Transference will occur, and unmet narcissistic demands will have consequences on group dynamics, regardless of the therapist's explanation of those behaviors.) Wittenberg (1975) discussed the pros and cons of the psychodynamic approach including use of confrontation with the adolescent substance-abusing population. She found that an art workshop approach with scanty interpretation of the art was beneficial for residential treatment adolescents who were already immersed in verbal therapy. Donnenberg (1978) described the impact of mural making in a substance abuse therapeutic community on group dynamics, including power struggles, scapegoating, and cohesiveness.

Virshup (1985) found that a weekly group art-therapy workshop that combined a string art technique with journaling and sharing enabled methadone clinic clients to communicate feelings and conflicts with each other, develop social skills, gain insight, and improve self-esteem. Feen-Calligan, Washington, and Moxley (2008) described the use of a visual-processing modality as a treatment component for a group of minority women in SAT. Participants responded to fine art reproductions chosen specifically by the researchers to enhance the therapeutic experience, by enabling access to emotions and stimulating recall of repressed areas. The participants seemed to benefit on a deep level by sharing responses to pre-chosen fine art reproductions that depicted the feminine experience; the cohesiveness of the group was enhanced by the universality of the themes.

Fernandez (2009) described a protocol for comic drawing in a group setting that provided clients with reflective distance and helped them explore ambivalence toward recovery. Sessions began with the development of a cartoon representation of their drinking/using self, progressed through a depiction of their recovery self, and then involved specific drawing tasks that combined these selves with various situations or environments. Skeffington and Browne (2014) discussed how an art therapy group allowed deeper self-disclosure for a woman whose initial presentation was reluctant. A key element in the group's success was the ability to allow the group behaviors and art products to inform an intuitive, rather than preconceived, approach by the therapist. Cox and Price (1990) described how their incident drawing directive (*draw an incident that occurred during the time when you were using*) enabled a decrease in defensiveness and encouraged feedback among adolescents participating in group art therapy for substance abuse.

Special topics for art therapy and addictions
Expressive Therapies Continuum
Hinz (2009a) created an elegant framework for assessing and treating substance abuse clients that builds on Kagin and Lusebrink's Expressive Therapies Continuum (ETC) (1978). Hinz's model links functions associated with levels of the ETC to addiction-specific characteristics

and needs, and provides corresponding interventions and directives. She recommends individualizing art therapy treatment plans based on ETC-based assessment. Group art therapists can physically lay out the range of available media along the continuum of fluid to resistant, and educate the group about media properties (2009b). Participants' choice of media provides an additional assessment marker. Lounsbury's (2015) dynamic weekly protocol coordinates tasks using pertinent media choices with the ETC, and is additionally linked to the client's location on the Stages of Change (SOC). The theme or content for the week's art work progresses through a list of the Twelve Step Principles (a.k.a. the Twelve Virtues), which are one-word themes correlated to the Twelve Steps.

Developmental and maturity issues

Moschini (2005) described the use of a developmental model when working with "difficult clients." Phases of therapy may be seen as paralleling the phases of development into a more mature identity. Moschini suggested specific art therapy interventions to complement the tasks of the eight Eriksonian stages of life. Matto *et al.* (2003) reported on the use of metaphor in art therapy to explore an adolescent client's personal fable, which involved perceived immunity to the effects of addiction. Groterath (1999) described how many addicts feel uncomfortable on the "stage of words" that may remind them of failure or inadequacy in a classroom or courtroom situation (p.21). Verbal therapies tend to re-enact such situations, inciting transference, with the counselor replacing the teacher or judge as the authority figure. By contrast, an art therapist is more likely to be seen as a peer or helper than an authority.

Morse *et al.* (2015) paired a Ladder of Change developmental model with corresponding arts activities as a basis for measurement of growth toward independence in SAT users. The ladder's bottom rung represented being stuck, isolated, and emotional; continuing upward, the steps progressed through wanting to be in others' company; sharing and engaging; and finally becoming self-reliant, relaxed, and helpful to others. Ten museum outreach sessions included participant involvement in murals, photography, digital storytelling, and other arts-based activities. Improvement was seen in levels of confidence, sociability, and wellbeing; Morse *et al.* recommend this approach as helpful for building resilience, maturity, and recovery capital.

Feelings and anxiety

"Feelings work" is a customary component in addiction treatment programming. Intentionally or not, substance abusers have suppressed their emotions through their substance abuse. Art therapy and art tasks may enable expression, containment, and an improved comfort level with feelings. The usefulness of art making in working with emotions is readily apparent, even to treatment providers who are otherwise unfamiliar with the benefits of art therapy. Foulke and Keller (1976) described a therapeutic community serving veterans who had been heroin addicts. They believed art therapy assisted the clients in "owning" their feelings, particularly those that they feared expressing in other ways. By externalizing feelings into imagery, participants could more easily link them to cognitions and verbal expressions. Forrest (1975) described a substance-abusing client who received art therapy at a psychiatric day hospital for eleven months following an overdose. This client opened up in response to Forrest's Rogerian manner—art making seemed to create a nonthreatening atmosphere and stimulate his ability to share his feelings verbally as well as in the art.

Manley (2014) found a reduction in anxiety in a small sample of patients ($n=15$) in a detoxification facility after doing a mandala intervention, even after controlling for drug of choice and length of stay on the unit. Laurer and van der Vennet (2015) researched the effect on negative mood and anxiety of 28 adults with SUD assigned to either an art production or image-sorting task. Statistical analysis indicated that length of time over treatment was the significant factor in the post-test reduction of negative mood.

Shame and trauma

According to Wilson (2012), SAT that focuses on practical approaches such as cognitive therapy may not address issues of shame, whereas art therapy could bypass intellectual and verbal defenses to access shame. In particular, Wilson proposed using art therapy to enhance shame reduction by exploring family-of-origin messages, addressing perfectionism and the need for control, and affirming a positive self-image. L. Johnson (1990) described fear of exposure of the shame-based self as an obstacle to spiritual rebirth and recovery, but stated that "creativity is an antidote to shame" in that it connects us to a higher creative power and to our true selves (p. 307).

Horovitz (2009) described working with a Deaf woman whose substance abuse and shame were compounded by her deafness and a history of being sexually abused. This client's gradual recovery was enabled by her creation of symbolic clay structures that allowed communication with the art therapist about abuse history that had previously been kept secret. Glover (1999) wrote specifically about substance abuse clients with a history of incest victimization and how the typical low self-esteem in a substance abuse client is even lower in this sub-population. The likelihood for failure in treatment is increased in programs that feature a confrontational or shaming approach, but play and arts therapies can provide a form of expression and release that improves the odds for recovery.

Spiritual, existential, and archetypal themes

Art therapists have observed the usefulness of art therapy to enable spiritual, existential, or archetypal exploration and healing for people with addiction issues (PWAI). Chickerneo (1993) used a heuristic inquiry to study the personal stories, art, art therapy process, and spirituality of people in recovery from substance abuse and codependency. Hagens (2011) used a grounded theory approach to explore the art expressions of women who had relapsed and returned to treatment. Strengths observed in the women's visual journals included positive use of the Twelve Step Principles and slogans, and individual definitions of higher power. Trust in the therapist was enabled by her familiarity with these concepts. Hagens suggested that creative arts approaches might serve as an alternative to Twelve Step work for some clients.

The practice of refraining from interpretation or analysis was emphasized by Feen-Calligan (1995) when she explored how art enables spiritual development, both through the creative act and through contemplation of the artwork. She designed a *doing by not doing* group for an inpatient addiction treatment program wherein no verbal processing was allowed. Clients were shown basic art techniques, then encouraged to relax, turn attention inward, and draw, paint, or sculpt as desired. Clients reported benefits from this restful space, which was in contrast to the rigor and verbal demands of the rest of the program.

Use of imagery has long been part of shamanic practice as well as of established religion. Allen (1985) showed slides of iconic paintings in SAT, engendering group discussion of existential issues that deepened participants' insight into their own lives. Colgate (2016) created a set of mixed-media art cards on foam core board that provided stimulus imagery and themes for clients to process resistance to change. Individual cards represent shadow themes within four suits (see Figures 1.1 and 1.2). Clients' projection of personal shadow issues onto the cards allowed them to be discussed more readily; in addition to verbal exploration, clients could journal, create response art, or make their own cards.

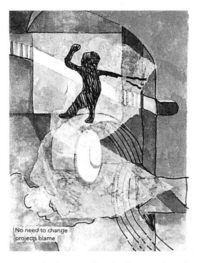

Figure 1.1: Shadow card. Suit: "No need to change." Card: "Projects blame" (see color plate)

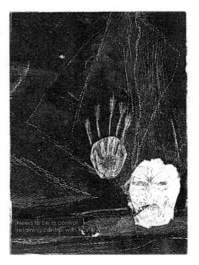

Figure 1.2: Shadow card. Suit: "Need to be in control." Card: "Retaining control with hostility" (see color plate)

Feen-Calligan's (1999) grounded theory study involved interviews with art therapists and psychiatrists working in addictions, and individuals in recovery; *enlightenment* emerged as a key concept describing the impact of art therapy in SAT (1999). Factors in the definition of enlightenment included self-insight, self-expression, and a natural high. Value was placed on the capacity of art making to be simultaneously playful, energizing, soothing, and relieving, or "en-lightening."

The Twelve Steps

Several art therapists have written about spirituality and the Twelve Steps in recovery from addictions. D.R. Johnson (1990) stated that while both insight-oriented psychotherapy and creative arts therapies help clients feel better about themselves, they may not be specific enough to be effective primary treatment for addiction. He advocated for arts therapies to align specifically with the Twelve Steps, such as by helping clients explore their own understanding of "god." He identified other specific issues that could be addressed this way: overcoming denial and shame (Step 1); imaging one's higher power (Step 2); depicting strengths and weaknesses (Step 4); and creating community-based arts activities (Step 12).

Julliard (1995) conducted research to increase chemically dependent patients' belief in Step 1 (admitting powerlessness over addiction) through art therapy and role-play. Change as measured by the research tool did not reach significance, but post-study interviews with the clients indicated their perception that their denial had lessened. His 1999 monograph discussed the Twelve Steps and ways in which art therapy and group work can support step work in a treatment setting. Krebs (2008) tested a 12-session protocol wherein a treatment group used each of four media (collage, drawing, clay, and painting) to respond to the first three steps. By reflecting on a single step on four occasions with a different media each time, clients experienced a more meaningful and satisfying engagement with each theme. Art therapists Nobis (2010) and Hayes (2012) created workbooks that provide specific art directives for each of the Twelve Steps.

Conclusion
Summary of benefits
Many of the authors cited in this chapter have identified ways in which art therapy meets the needs of the SAT population. Mahony (1999) summarized the beneficial functions of art therapy for those with SUD as:

- facilitating expression of repressed or complicated emotions
- protecting as well as uncovering defenses
- providing containment of shame, anguish, and rage
- enabling feelings of control through distancing
- identifying strengths to counteract feelings of inadequacy
- reducing isolation through improved communication and symbolic expression

(adapted from Mahony 1999, pp.118–119)

The chapters that follow in this book will support and illustrate these and other concepts.

Commentary on the status of art therapy in substance abuse treatment
Currently and individually, the fields of art therapy and addiction are experiencing excitement over neurological research findings. The idea that art therapists could elucidate a stand-alone approach to treating addiction (e.g., using art making to replace the function of drug use in the neurological reward pathway) might be compared to the pharmaceutical industry's dream of developing a universal cure for addiction. But broader research still supports a multidimensional approach to the treatment of addiction (NIDA 2012). I hope that in our zeal for the latest scientific findings, we do not lose sight of art therapy's remarkable versatility and the myriad ways in which this can be demonstrated.

I disagree with the idea (overheard at an art therapy conference session on addiction) that because experimental proof of art therapy's effectiveness is needed, we should not be "wasting time telling stories." Research is needed that demonstrates the proficiency of art therapy on *all* of the healing dimensions for addictions, from brain function to aesthetic and spiritual experience. A deep understanding of art therapy requires different ways of knowing, and I would venture that much of what is or will be proven by neurological research has been known in more intuitive (and often richer) ways for much longer. The challenge for art therapy researchers is, as Gerber wrote in support of mixed methods, to find "approaches that possess the necessary validity, trustworthiness, rigor, and creativity to satisfy the dominant culture while simultaneously preserving the philosophical and theoretical integrity of the field" (2016, p.654).

For clinicians who are attempting to convince established treatment providers of the benefits of art therapy, stories and anecdotal examples are a powerful, time-honored means of marketing, educating, and leaving a lasting impression. It is not unusual for dually certified art therapists to qualify for a job via their counseling credential, and then to hope to incorporate art therapy into an established program regimen. The provision of sample groups, working with volunteer clients individually and sharing client testimonials with agency administration, is more likely to succeed in this aim than citing scientific research for an art-therapy-based approach to treating addiction (if it existed). At the local level, pictures and stories are an effective starting place for getting the attention of employers who have already implemented the established best practices in their field. While I do honor the researchers who seek to build scientific evidence of the value of our profession, I also honor the clinicians who are using the art and stories to help people receiving treatment and to educate others who are stakeholders in addiction treatment.

If the preceding look at our literature has not already done so, I intend that the coming pages will convince the reader of the value of art therapy as a versatile addition to all aspects of addiction treatment. I hope this book will also supply a foundation of knowledge that will stimulate a desire to learn more, by reading, networking with other professionals, pursuing academic or continuing education opportunities, and perhaps by performing research. Armed with an understanding of both fields and a creative mindset, art therapists can effectively help people seeking recovery from addiction.

2

Substance Abuse Theory and Drugs of Abuse

This chapter reviews definitions of addiction and the two currently dominant models, the medical model, which lately has been informed by neuroscience research, and the biopsychosocial (BPS) model. These two conceptions of addiction do not negate one another, but treatment approaches may vary depending on which is dominant at a particular setting. A case vignette of art therapy with a person with alcohol use disorder and chronic post-traumatic stress disorder (PTSD) is described by making reference to neuroscience concepts and art therapy concepts such as those of the Expressive Therapies Continuum (ETC). The chapter concludes with basic information about substances of abuse.

Defining addiction: disease and behavior

In the late 1930s in the US, when an experiment in national prohibition of alcohol had failed and alcoholism was considered to involve a condition of hopeless moral bankruptcy, in his preface to the book *Alcoholics Anonymous* (AA 2001, first published 1939), physician William Silkworth identified it as a chronic disease. Alcoholics Anonymous (AA) cofounder Bill Wilson described alcoholism as an illness most akin to an allergy: he had correctly surmised that some people are inherently more susceptible than others to the condition. Alcoholism has been included in medical disease categorizations since the mid-20th century by the World Health Organization (WHO) and the American Medical Association (AMA) (Stevens and Smith 2013, first published 1998).

Since that era, understandings of the brain have contributed to the evidence that alcohol and other drugs (AOD) addiction is a disease by the standard definition in that it creates a progressive dysfunction in a particular part of the body (the brain, and in particular, the nucleus accumbens) that produces predictable, observable symptoms (McCauley 2009). The American Society of Addiction Medicine (ASAM 2011) defines addiction as a primary, chronic, and relapsing brain disease characterized by the pathological pursuit of reward and/or relief by substance use. In essence, the brain is altered by the addiction in ways that promote the continuance of the substance-using behavior. As with diseases like diabetes, asthma, and heart disease, the etiology of addiction involves genetics, environmental influences, and behavioral choices; also similarly, with successful management, death or disability from the disease may be avoided (Heilig 2015). Government research has shown that treatment relapse rates for drug addiction (40–60 percent) fall between those for diabetes (30–50 percent) and hypertension or asthma (50–70 percent) (NIDA 2015). Still, the general public, and even many professionals working in treatment and medicine, struggle to view addiction as a disease.

As with other diseases, long-term management does not equate to a cure. Those in long-term abstinence may show no outward signs of having an addiction, and a return to use may initially be manageable, but before long the amount used, physical tolerance, and BPS consequences are back to the former problematic level (Faulkner 2013; Mooney, Dold, and Eisenberg 2014). Some chronic alcohol users who relapse in later life find that their once-high biological tolerance has peaked and declined, and they are no longer capable of managing even token amounts of the drug.

Substance abuse and brain function

The brain's natural reward function involves the release of the neurotransmitter dopamine in the nucleus accumbens, known informally as the brain's pleasure center, which results in feelings of wellbeing or bliss. This action occurs in response to experiences or behaviors that support the individual or human evolution, such as social cues, food, and sexual activity. By their pharmacological action, all addictive drugs also create a release of dopamine, which may be more intense than that produced by natural rewards (Trafton and

Gifford 2008). In addition, some drugs affect other neurotransmitters. A typical pharmacological action is that the addictive drug plugs the reuptake site for the pleasure-causing neurotransmitter, which allows it to flood the channels between neurons and repeatedly stimulate them. In this action, it is not the drug itself that is making the person high, but the overabundance of dopamine. The type of drug will create particular effects such as sedating or stimulating the central nervous system, or affecting other neurotransmitters such as gabapentin or serotonin, which contributes (among other factors, such as individual differences and the using environment) to the sense of different highs for different drugs (Capuzzi and Stauffer 2016).

Repeated drug use results in dopamine neurons firing twice, the first time at any predictive cue (called a *trigger* in the treatment setting) that has been learned, and again, on impact of the drug's chemical action on the brain. Thus, for the habitual user, substance use cues will reinforce behavior more strongly than habitual natural reward cues, for which dopamine firing occurs only once (Trafton 2015). In time, a person who previously would have experienced pleasure at playing with their child or making love with a spouse will now have a flatter response to these activities. The artificial high brought on by drugs and the double firing to which the brain has become accustomed has created a new "normal" that cannot be matched by previously rewarding activities.

As an addicted person continues to use the drug, tolerance is acquired, and the artificial high becomes flatter as well. In a natural attempt to achieve homeostasis, the brain has started to produce less dopamine in response to what it perceives as overstock. Now when the person tries to stop use of the drug, natural chemicals are depleted, mood is even lower than the original normal state (which for some people was already depressed), and formerly pleasurable nondrug-related activities have no appeal (Capuzzi and Stauffer 2016; Trafton and Gifford 2008).

Meantime, predictive cues or triggers for drug use have become entrenched. Relapse potential exists whenever a recovering person encounters anything—"people, places, or things," as is said in AA—associated with former use, including everyday items such as mirrors or spoons that were used in drug preparation, or idiosyncratic reminders like a certain street corner. These triggering events involve neural responses to sensorily delivered cues that will fade as the brain heals (Mooney *et al.* 2014). For example, someone who has recently quit smoking cigarettes may feel mildly euphoric when encountering the smell of cigarette smoke; the feeling dissipates quickly when not followed by actual ingestion of the chemical. A period of time after quitting, the person finds the same odor has become neutral or unpleasant: it is no longer a predictive cue that releases dopamine.

Pharmaceutical approaches to treatment

Despite recent advances in psycho-pharmacological treatment, which are occasionally hailed in the popular press as "cures" for addiction, pharmaceutical treatment alone is insufficient for comprehensive or sustained recovery (Mendenhall 2014). Recovery from dopamine depletion or synaptic damage caused by addiction is most effectively accomplished by abstinence, healthy physical and social habits, and time (Mooney *et al.* 2014). Neuroscience is also providing evidence that brain plasticity and recovery is enhanced by relational attachment and the firing of mirror neurons, which lends scientific support to the intuitively derived founding theories of AA that are based on the benefits of fellowship (Capuzzi and Stauffer 2016; Nuckols 2016).

Of course, patience, employing healthy new habits, engaging in a Twelve Steps fellowship, and refraining from temptations to relapse are not an appealing protocol for most people. This is one reason that modern pharmacological approaches can be an important addition to a treatment regimen. Clients are assisted to withstand the brain-based drive to return to substance use until psychosocial and other treatments can take hold. Some clients will view the pharmacological treatment as a permanent necessity, whereas others will seek the ultimate goal of needing neither the illicit drug nor the pharmacological treatment (Trafton 2015).

One type of pharmacological treatment frequently used for heroin includes opioid *agonists* or partial agonists, such as methadone or buprenorphine, that block withdrawal symptoms and reduce cravings without providing the heroin high. An alternative type of treatment is an *antagonist* drug such as naltrexone, which blocks the action of drugs on the brain, so that a person will not get high if they relapse, and may even suffer adverse reactions. Naltrexone has been demonstrated as effective with opioids and alcohol; disulfiram (marketed as Antabuse) is a well-known antagonist drug used to treat alcohol addiction. Dedication and motivation are necessary to take a daily dose of an antagonist prescription; it is tempting to go off the prescription in order to enjoy a binge weekend. A monthly injectable form of naltrexone was developed to minimize this problem (Willey 2016).

Pharmaceuticals such as selective serotonin reuptake inhibitors (SSRIs) and other antidepressants are often used for those in early recovery. Anhedonia is a particular problem for people recovering from stimulants like methamphetamine and cocaine, and antidepressants may be beneficial in the short term. This class of treatment may also be indicated for those with comorbid presentations of depression, anxiety, or chronic PTSD (Willey 2016). As recovery progresses, it is best practice for the prescribing professional to adjust this type of prescription based on ongoing diagnostic assessment to identify whether depression, anxiety, or other comorbid symptoms were an underlying condition of the substance use, or a result. Art therapists may be able to assist with ongoing assessment by comparing art products of a client produced during the acute and post-acute withdrawal period.

Art therapists working in this field should be knowledgeable of all treatment options offered to their clients, and be supportive of individualized treatment choices that include a variety of techniques. Broad-based approaches that make use of a variety of treatment modalities are recommended by addiction research teams funded by the US government (NIDA 2012, 2015) as well as by other professionals (Mendenhall 2014; Trafton 2015; Willey 2016).

Art therapy through a neuroscience lens

Several art therapists have described the beneficial functions of art therapy within the framework of clinical neuroscience; a few relevant principles are outlined in the following, and exemplified in my work with Heidi. Although knowledge of neuroscience is not required to provide art therapy in SAT, it provides another useful lens for describing how art therapy works in general, or in a specific case.

A basic understanding of anatomy informs this topic. The central nervous system consists of the brain and spinal cord, and affects the rest of the body via the peripheral nervous system. The latter consists of the sympathetic nervous system, which responds to stress in the environment, and the parasympathetic nervous system, which enables a return to a more relaxed state. Mind-body approaches to health or healing, such as biofeedback and mindfulness meditation, involve rebalancing the sympathetic and parasympathetic systems to reduce stress. Another part of the peripheral nervous system, the somatic system, manages voluntary muscle responses to incoming sensory messages. Art therapy may involve both these systemic functions. Clients can experience relief from stress by experiencing kinesthetic and sensory pleasure through physical control over art media and products (Hass-Cohen and Carr 2008).

The function of working with the hands has been shown to provide stress relief. The nucleus accumbens or pleasure center interfaces with motor and cognitive functions. So-called "effort-driven rewards" are achieved by successful involvement with activities that require coordinating hand and mind to meet a challenge (Lambert 2008). The satisfaction provided by this kind of work is an excellent replacement for drug activation of the same neurotransmitters. Chapter 6 provides further discussion of using art activities to engage the flow state.

Art therapy also offers communicative functions for healing. Particularly in infancy, but also throughout the lifespan, the brain changes and grows in response to social-emotional communications. Affect regulation is determined by connectivity between various parts of the brain, which are arranged in a developmental hierarchy. Basic emotions emerging from the lower parts of the brain, the amygdala, and limbic system are regulated in the higher brain region of the cortex. Within the cortex, some specialization occurs within lobes of the left and right hemispheres, with verbal processing reaching a peak in the left. During times of stress or crisis, brain functioning reverts to the survival mode processes of the limbic system; the experience of fear or anger may dominate and prohibit the modulating effect of cortical thinking (Hass-Cohen and Carr 2008). When people are in a crisis state, they may be unable to mentally assign words to their experience at all, let alone to utter them (Hull 2002). However, art therapy can operate without the verbal function by enabling emotional expression through sensory and symbolic communication. The Expressive Therapies Continuum (ETC) can lend guidance to a developmental approach to healing brain functioning that has been derailed by trauma and addiction (Hinz 2009b).

The case of Heidi

Having experienced severely traumatic events as an adult and throughout her childhood, Heidi battled chronic anxiety, depression, and PTSD. Working with a team of independent outpatient providers (a psychiatrist for medication management, a psychologist for talk therapy, and myself for art therapy), she had made significant gains in addressing past trauma. However, she had come to rely on wine as a coping mechanism, and realized that this was becoming problematic.

As for many trauma survivors, everyday life experiences could be difficult for Heidi, especially at times when she was having an increase of stress or flashbacks. An event such as being pushed accidently from behind while standing in line could trigger panic. Heidi and I had established a strong therapeutic relationship, and she considered my studio to be one of few places where she felt totally safe. When she would arrive for a session unable to speak, we made use of art therapy to help her self-regulate. She chose materials from the range of studio supplies, and her choices would often, intentionally or not, have a communicative property. She frequently made use of the art materials at a kinesthetic-sensory level, which engaged the regulating aspects of the somatic and parasympathetic systems; she also performed at a higher cortical level when she engaged in symbolization, which allowed her to communicate even when she had no words.

In one such silent session, she did nothing but repeatedly and deliberately form white plasticine balls around orange pony beads. She seemed to be making protective casings for vulnerable, penetrable self-objects; the orange color was one she had previously assigned to her incest experience, and her personally established motif of a white cloud or nest, sometimes tied to the ability to dissociate, represented serenity, escape, and safety. The power of this session was quite humbling. I simply served as a silent witness to her performance of this protective, perseverative ritual, and she needed me for that very function; yet I struggled with the absence of verbal processing and wished for a magic wand to speed passage of this strange wordless therapy. We later discussed that session's effectiveness, both as an action that enabled her to regain self-control, and as an experience that created a deeper bond between us, for she trusted me to sit there and allow her to do what was needed. She knew I would not enforce my power over her by being directive when that was contraindicated by her coming into the studio and demonstrating her own solution.

In addition, I gained empathy for her in a way that I could not have, had we been forcing verbal processing.

In another nonverbal session, having chosen soft oil pastels as her medium, she spent the therapy hour creating a white rectangle that was grounded on the page bottom and encased on the other three sides by a thick blue boundary. She was greatly agitated at first, but seemed to be self-soothing by stroking the creamy white pastel repeatedly to make the box, and building up the deep blue pastel into a thick wall. It seemed I could literally feel anxiety, rage, and despair disseminating out into the air between us via this white portal. I have used this drawing as a teaching tool because it demonstrates the often invisible function of overtly primitive imagery: anyone viewing this drawing without its appended label would find it meaningless, but it emitted absolute power during its making and witnessing. Before she left, Heidi silently labeled the drawing "SAFE PLACE."

At the following session, vocal again, Heidi explained the impetus for that drawing: her grandmother, who was aware of the incest history and still insisted on trying to make a happy family, had walked into Heidi's house unannounced to try to talk her into coming to a family dinner. Heidi had felt utterly violated and furious at this sudden infiltration of her safe home space. With the bounded box drawing, she had been self-soothing as well as symbolically creating a new, unspoiled, and inviolable home space. The safe place theme was perpetually helpful for her, and she had regulated her feelings at the limbic level by creating a sensorily soothing version of it the previous week. Now we were able to process the situation verbally, at the level of the cortex, again, in the safe space of our relationship in the studio.

Although Heidi had no particular art experience or ability, she effectively used art and craft materials as a way to express her most raw and wordless feelings. Her brain was perceiving the art making as a reward activity, and she herself volunteered the idea that she could make art instead, when she felt compelled to pour a glass of wine. She purchased her own supply of materials, and created a special area in her home where she could make altered books and collages or work with clay. Sometimes she would work on a sensory level; other times she worked more intentionally to express emotion; or she would work on a verbal analytic level by adding titles, labels, or poetry, or bringing a project to me to discuss. Although she was not familiar with the ETC, she seemed to be employing it to full benefit.

For in-home art making to serve as a substitute activity for her drinking, Heidi realized she would need to maintain a healthy boundary around preserving a personal art space in her home. Occasionally, on her own terms, she opened the space to her children so they could enjoy making things together. She also shared some of her finished work with her husband, which increased his empathy for her chronic emotional experience. Family activities that centered on art making and processing provided additional relational healing.

Art making is not a direct substitute for a beloved drug, in that it will not provide the additional pharmaceutical release of dopamine. However, as biological dependence on a drug is removed, art making and relational activities can become a preferred substitute for stress relief. The art making is not just relaxing in the sense of being a distracting activity, such as watching TV; it is a proactive, mind-hand endeavor that promotes the flow state and resultant wellbeing. Heidi's increased willingness to share positive bonding experiences with her family also promoted neurological healing via reparative attachment experiences.

The biopsychosocial model

The establishment of addiction as a disease is important for parity in research funding, treatment applications, and insurance coverage. It is also important to teach to people in treatment, as it helps relieve internalized shame, stigma, and guilt. However, addiction should not be viewed as a purely brain-based condition. Etiological theories of addiction and recovery have rightly shifted over time from moral explanations to medical models. But just as we acknowledge that characterological identity does not come wholly from either genetics or the environment, a BPS conceptualization of addiction is believed to be most helpful for understanding individual clients' etiology and for guiding treatment.

The BPS model is used to discuss etiology and clinical applications in medicine, allied health, mental health, and sociology. In addiction treatment, spirituality is sometimes considered a fourth factor (BPSS); alternatively, existential or transpersonal issues might be included in the psychological area, or religious community in the social. The BPS model probably originated in the 1970s with the psychiatrist George Engel, who sought an alternative to the purely "medical model" of physical and mental disease that was then in vogue. He believed that many factors other than biological or medical ones contributed to both the etiology and treatment of diseases and disorders. As an example, a heart patient's chronic untreated depression leads to inability to lose weight, which aggravates his medical condition; upon experiencing heart pain, his personality is such that he denies it; within his social environment, a knowledgeable work mate insists he seek emergency treatment; junior staff at the emergency room (ER) do not administer proper procedure and he suffers an irreversible change to his condition; and so forth. A purely medical description of this patient's heart condition might be accurate, but would have limited value in identifying important factors for a comprehensive treatment plan (Engel 1977).

In a similar manner, the BPS model can be used to understand differences in drug effects. The phenomenological experience of any particular instance of drug-taking will vary depending on the dynamic interaction of three variables; the *agent*, or drug itself, its pharmacological action, potency, etc. (bio); the *host*, or qualities of the person taking the drug, such as whether they have underlying depression, are tired, or anticipate a certain type of high (psycho); and the *environment*, which includes factors that can influence the experience such as a nightclub setting or being with certain other people (social).

When a clinician has observed the variety of clinical presentations involved with addiction, it is difficult to deny the impact of biological, psychological, behavioral, and environmental variables on the underlying brain-based disease. So, while it is striking that there are still those who are unable to view addiction as a disease, it is also striking that there are those who insist that addiction is *purely* a biological condition. Discussion of these issues is important to the treatment process. Learning about the biological basis of addiction helps to relieve shame and reinforce the importance of abstinence. Teaching clients about the other BPS variables and encouraging them to identify their own unique mix of these factors are enlightening and encourage personal investment in designing a treatment and recovery plan. To meet the needs of a psychoeducational curriculum, I developed a therapeutic graphic art activity with an informational handout about the BPS that is particularly beneficial when processed in groups (see Appendix A). Each client's chart reveals a unique mix, but also reflects the universal factors of this multifaceted disease.

Using this accessible activity, clients more readily understand and discuss the factors involved in their addiction, which in turn informs recovery planning.

Drugs of abuse: pharmacology and select current issues

This section provides a brief overview of the primary substances of abuse. Readers who are new to the field of substance abuse are urged to learn more from reliable sources, such as those given in Appendix B. All those who work with this population will want to stay current about social policy, research, and the latest drugs to appear on the streets or online. This section emphasizes current issues pertaining to opioid use, which has reached epidemic status in the US.

Depressants

Depressants are a broad classification of drugs including sedatives and opioids that depress the central nervous system "from the top down," beginning with the prefrontal cortex. For example, someone who is drinking will first feel disinhibited; then judgment is compromised and risks are taken that would not be otherwise; next, reaction time, vision, and balance become affected; physical effects proceed to incoherence, staggering, and loss of consciousness. If enough is ingested in a short enough time, coma and death can result. With all the depressants, physical tolerance develops, which means the same amount of drug becomes less effective over time. This poses a problem for ongoing prescription use; at a certain point, the drugs are no longer effective at the level prescribed, but continually increasing the dose would be deadly.

Withdrawal from depressants entails the brain striving to come back to balance. This will initially involve the opposite of sedation, or agitation, which is expressed in withdrawal or hangover symptoms such as shaking, headaches, and jitteriness. Seizures and hallucinations are common in withdrawal from long-term habitual use of alcohol and benzodiazepines; withdrawal from these types of drugs can be deadly and should be medically managed for chronic users. Withdrawal from opioids involves severe body pains, cramps, nausea, and diarrhea. Although it is a miserable experience, it is not life threatening unless the person is also withdrawing from alcohol or other sedatives or has other health complications (Smith 2013).

Alcohol and other sedatives

Chemically named ethanol, alcohol is the most widely abused psychotropic substance, and it produces the most problems for society in terms of medical expense, lost productivity, accidents, associated crime, and damage to families (Stevens and Smith 2013). The fact that alcohol is legal for adults does not mean that it is not a problem for someone with an established addiction to substances; use of alcohol must be addressed even in clients who present with another drug of choice.

The amount of ethanol is approximately equivalent in a typical can or bottle of beer, glass of wine, or mixed drink. Clients may try to argue this point (usually beer drinkers believe beer to be a "lighter" beverage). They are also often misled by the fact of their own tolerance to alcohol. Being able to "hold one's liquor" or "drink everyone else under the table" is not a sign that the person is resistant to dependence, but rather that the disease has progressed because tolerance is in evidence. The experience of blackouts, or periods of time when the person was functioning but later has no memory of what occurred, is thought to be another early sign of physical dependence or a genetic predisposition to dependence. Blackouts indicate the user was able to ingest enough of the substance (any type of depressant, but most commonly alcohol) to interfere with brain consolidation of short-term memory, yet remain conscious and functional (Chamberlain 2013).

Other sedatives include barbiturates (such as prescription sleeping pills and anesthetics) and the anti-anxiety and anti-seizure medications or tranquilizers, including benzodiazepines (e.g., Xanax® and Klonopin®). Although most of these drugs are manufactured legally, they are also produced on the black market and are readily available on the streets. GHB and Rohypnol® are frequently abused sedatives that may be used in conjunction with a stimulant drug to create a mellower, more euphoric high. They are also known as "date rape drugs" because they are used to facilitate sexual assault. Slipping the drug into a victim's alcoholic drink renders the person cooperative and usually also induces a blackout.

Opioids

Opioids is a general term that covers synthetic and naturally derived painkillers. *Opiates* refers to the subcategory of opioids that is naturally derived from the opium poppy, which includes smokable opium, morphine, and heroin. Pharmacologically, these depressant drugs may be referred to as narcotics or narcotic analgesics, in reference to their soporific and painkilling effects. Outside the medical or scientific arena, the term *narcotic* is sometimes used more broadly to mean illicit psychoactive drugs; for example, in law enforcement, marijuana may be referred to as a narcotic (Kuhn, Swartzwelder, and Wilson 2014).

Because of the current epidemic use of opioids, therapists working in substance abuse should be aware of the sociopolitical issues around these drugs. In the earlier part of this century, the trend in the pharmaceutical industry was to actively promote more varieties and ever-more-potent versions of painkilling drugs, which resulted in a higher percentage of people being prescribed and becoming addicted to them. Sales of prescription pain relievers in 2010 were four times those ten years earlier (CDC 2014). In 2012 in the US, 259 million prescriptions were written for opioids, which was more than enough to give every adult in the country a bottle of pills (SAMHSA 2016).

Illicit trade in pharmaceuticals has expanded both in the streets and online. Legitimate prescribers are now becoming more wary of offering and automatically refilling prescriptions. This at least partially explains the fact that 94 percent of respondents in a 2014 survey of people in treatment for opioid addiction said they began to buy heroin instead of their prescription painkiller (despite the fact that heroin is not sold legally) because prescription opioids had become "far more expensive and harder to obtain" (Cicero *et al.* 2014, p.824). It is estimated that four in five new heroin users first misused prescription painkillers (Jones 2013). These facts underscore the need for pain management to be addressed in recovery. Art therapists can take advantage of the function of art therapy to reduce the perception of physical pain. Art therapy is sometimes also cited as a mind-body or alternative health approach along with mindfulness training, yoga, and other approaches that are also being used to manage chronic pain (Angheluta and Lee 2011).

Stimulants

Drugs that stimulate the central nervous system are as addictive as depressants, although this was not always thought to be so. Those who are chronic users may experience tolerance and progression of symptoms that include paranoia and psychosis. Withdrawal from stimulants is uncomfortable but not medically deadly. The greatest difficulty for those attempting to establish sobriety from stimulants is the long-lasting malaise and anhedonia that is a result of severe depletion of the brain's naturally occurring feel-good chemicals (such as dopamine) (Mooney *et al.* 2014).

Legal stimulants include energy drinks, caffeine pills, and nicotine; prescription medications include those used to treat attention deficit hyperactivity disorder (ADHD), being overweight, and sleep disorders (e.g., Ritalin®, Adderall®, and Dexedrine®). These drugs are often sold or traded outside a prescription (Streetdrugs.org 2016).

Stimulant use has been popular among teens and college students for decades. Off-prescription stimulants or over-the-counter products like NoDoz® or energy drinks are taken to counteract the sedative effects of alcohol or other drugs so the person can party longer or stay up and study. This trend did not go unnoticed by alcoholic beverage manufacturers, and now canned drinks known as CABs (caffeinated alcoholic beverages) or AEDs (alcoholic energy drinks) are available in sweetened formulations with marketing geared toward young people. It is estimated that approximately one-third of people aged 12–24 use these drinks on a regular basis. In some of these canned beverages, the alcohol content is over twice that found in beer. The product creates a "wide-awake drunk"—the user doesn't perceive that they are impaired by alcohol, but actually may be dangerously so (NCADD 2015).

Methamphetamine

Methamphetamine, also known as meth, crystal, or crank, is a strong stimulant that has euphoric qualities but can also provoke irritable or aggressive behavior. Meth is readily made in portable illicit labs; improper procedure and storage can accidently result in chemical explosions. Meth is usually sold on the streets as a powder that is snorted or mixed with water and injected. Meth that has been prepared as smokable chunks or rocks is known as *ice*. Chronic long-term users, who may rarely eat or sleep, are known for an appearance that includes rapid onset of aging, loss of teeth, and skin lesions, which are aggravated by dehydration and malnutrition. Tolerance to the drug and depletion of natural brain chemicals means that even when using, they are no longer able to feel passably okay. After learning about meth addiction in a psychoeducational group, Alicia drew an expressive picture of her "brain on meth" (see Figure 2.1). She wrote that it was "tangled up and full of black holes…parts that used to be happy are disconnected." Despite her negative written description, the drawing has a certain seductive appeal, perhaps reflective of the drug it references.

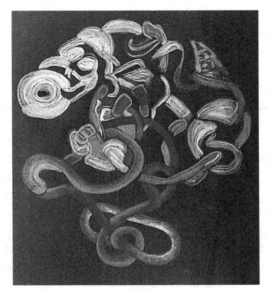

Figure 2.1: Alicia's "Brain on meth" (see color plate)

Cocaine

Cocaine is a white powder derived from the coca plant that is used intranasally or intravenously. *Crack* is a freebase version of cocaine sold in inexpensive small chunks or rocks and smoked in a pipe, which results in a more intense high. The high experienced in early stage cocaine use combines alert euphoria with an absolute sense of wellbeing and self-esteem. Cocaine and crack are often used in binge fashion, with the person *chasing the high*, using repeatedly as the previous dose wears off, until physically the body must *crash*. During a binge, the person usually goes without food or sleep, becomes increasingly irritable and restless, and may experience panic attacks, paranoia, and psychotic episodes (Streetdrugs.org 2016). Due to its rapid and intense high, crack is particularly addictive; relapse rates are high, and triggers and cravings are essential topics for treatment. As with other stimulant drugs like methamphetamine, anhedonia that results from brain depletion of neurotransmitters is a primary factor in relapse.

Marijuana

Marijuana, the common name for the plant cannabis sativa, is classified by itself because it is chemically very complex. Any given plant contains hundreds of biologically active chemicals that have diverse effects on various parts of the brain and body (Inaba 2015). Research has established helpful medical effects of nonpsychoactive chemicals found in marijuana (such as cannabidiol), as well as the harmful medical effects of the cannabinoids that are psychoactive (such as THC). It is not necessary to obtain the high in order to obtain the medical benefits, which include pain relief, immune system support, and anti-nausea and anti-seizure properties. Some medically useful cannabinoids are available in pill form and have been approved by the US Food and Drug Administration (FDA); others are still being researched. The FDA has not approved the marijuana plant for medical use (Streetdrugs.org 2016).

For decades, illicit growers have agriculturally engineered the marijuana plant itself to produce more of the euphoria-producing THC. In recent years, both licit and illicit marijuana product development has become a burgeoning business. In Colorado, where sales of recreational marijuana are legal, conventions are held wherein vendors vie to produce the most intense product. *Wax* or *dab* is intensely concentrated THC that appears as small bits of a golden brown wax-looking substance. *Dabbing* refers to inhaling the drug using a vaporizer or e-cigarette; users say that one hit is equivalent to smoking several joints of high-grade product (Streetdrugs.org 2016). *Spice* or *fake weed* is smokable plant material to which synthetic cannabinoids have been applied.

Marijuana is the drug most often listed as a problem by the over 1.8 million people treated each year for addiction in the US; this includes people who are multidrug users (Inaba 2015). Several sources of data support the estimate that approximately one-tenth of those who use marijuana will develop dependence and be unable to stop without treatment (NIDA 2013). This leaves a significant number who use it recreationally and protest its harmlessness; perhaps no other drug is so controversial in this way. As substance abuse counselors know well, even people whose use is obviously problematic are capable of endlessly citing fake news and unsubstantiated evidence in favor of marijuana use; some maintain an "ardent denial about it even being a drug" (Inaba 2015, p.22). Therapists may need to gently point out that websites such as www.gethigh.com are not run by impartial research institutes.

Arlene created a bridge drawing featuring trees that look like a harvested marijuana plant (see Figure 2.2). One member of her art therapy group who was familiar with bridge-drawing symbolism (and marijuana) suggested to her that this "good bud" appeared to be in her immediate future (right side of the bridge). Another quipped that the picture's title should be "happy little trees" in reference to the use of that term by a popular television landscape-painting instructor who was particularly mellow. Arlene's image, in conjunction with her repeated insistence that her drug of choice was natural and harmless, did not bode well for her prognosis. However, perhaps a wiser part of herself is depicted in the behavior of her dog, who she described as her closest friend. He appears to be leading her in the other direction, away from temptation.

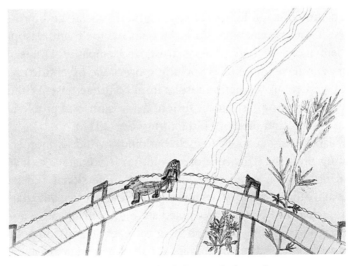

Figure 2.2: Arlene's "Happy little trees"

Use of marijuana results in the suppression of short-term memory, difficulty in problem-solving, and confusion when attempting to complete tasks that require multiple steps. With continued use, this loss of function impacts the ability to learn or to retain what is learned (Inaba 2015). After Arlene had started getting more honest with me, she confided that she had been high on marijuana for her first three years of college and was now terrified to try to finish her degree, because she could not remember a single thing she had studied. Many habitual marijuana users are also involved in other compulsive or isolating activities, such as video gaming, that further stall social development and the building of mature relationships. Arlene had lost friends who had tired of her continually stoned presentation; her dog had become her substitute for human intimacy.

Other substances of abuse

People abuse other types of drugs that are not clearly in the stimulant or depressant category, including hallucinogens, or psychedelics, which alter the user's perceptions of reality. This class of drug includes substances derived directly from plants, mushrooms, or fungi, as well as synthetics made in laboratories. Peyote, psilocybin (magic mushrooms), LSD, MDMA (ecstasy, Molly), ketamine (Special K) and others provide hallucinations, altered sensory perceptions, delusions, and disordered thinking. Ecstasy is particularly popular as a club drug due to one of its neurological functions that heightens social and pro-sexual feelings: it causes release of the hormones oxytocin and vasopressin, which enhances feelings of love, trust, and empathy. Drugs in this category can have dire effects, including paranoia, psychotic episodes, seizures, and coma. Addiction results from continued use. Withdrawal usually features long-lasting confusion, depression, and problems with sleep, attention, and memory (Streetdrugs.org 2016).

Off-label use of anabolic (muscle-building) steroids is another major illicit drug problem. This type of steroid has legitimate veterinary and medical uses, but is often used illegally by professional and amateur athletes and others who may obtain the drug from bootleg manufacturers. The drug does not provide an immediate high, but users on a regular regimen report feelings of euphoria, great energy, and competitive or combative feelings. Chronic users are at risk of heart damage and stroke; those who stop using experience depression (Kuhn *et al.* 2014).

Legal and treatment issues with new drugs

The continual development of new drugs in both regulated and illicit laboratories has been an increasing challenge to interdiction and regulation over the last 50 years. In the US, psychoactive drugs are listed in a regulatory schedule established by the Controlled Substances Act. Drugs are placed in one of five categories, ranging from those with established medical use and low abuse potential, often available over the counter (Schedule V), to those with high abuse potential and no established medical use, which are illegal (Schedule I) (Smith 2013).

Designer drugs are so called because chemists design them to be similar to drugs of abuse. Those with stimulant or psychedelic properties are often referred to as *club drugs* since they are frequently used in that environment. Drugs developed in illicit labs that act similarly to a prototype on the schedule may be perfectly legal because they are technically not included in the regulatory description. In addition, they may be identified or marketed in creative ways designed to avoid or minimize legal issues. For example, the term *bath salts* was originally the product label used to market various formulations of designer stimulant/hallucinogenic drugs in head shops and online (Streetdrugs.org 2016). An amendment to the Controlled Substances Act allows any drug with a chemical structure substantially similar to one already included to be temporarily banned for three years, allowing time for research to ascertain whether the ban should become permanent (Smith 2013). However, that process is cumbersome. A recent example of a harmful drug avoiding regulation is that of *Pink*, a new synthetic opioid estimated to be eight times stronger than heroin, which is sold online by overseas sources and in the streets. Although the Drug Enforcement Agency, which enforces the Controlled Substances Act, acted to have this product temporarily classified as a Category I substance, many confirmed deaths have occurred while the legal procedure for interdiction catches up with the legal availability of the drug (Partnership News Service 2016).

Opioids purchased on the street are particularly dangerous because unpredictable differences in potency can readily result in overdose (Smith 2013). The typical purchaser of street or illicit online drugs will never know for sure what they are buying. At the lower levels of drug dealing, particularly among adolescents, even the sellers may not know the identity of the drug they are peddling.

Conclusion

In response to a 2015 survey, 6.5 million Americans over the age of 12 reported using controlled prescription medicines nonmedically during the past month, which made this kind of illicit drug use second only to marijuana, and more than past-month use of heroin, cocaine, and hallucinogens combined (SAMHSA 2016). Knowledge of such trends and of current drugs of abuse is important for art therapists and other professionals; in essence, this is cultural knowledge. It might be compared, for example, to the need to learn about military culture and terminology in order to work with that population.

Client-supplied information can contradict that gained through professional sources and still be valid, due to individual differences (the interplay of agent, host, environment), local drug supply variations, or differences in local or regional slang. For example, the slang term "water" has been used to refer to a number of drugs that are not similar pharmacologically. Alternatively, client-supplied knowledge may be incorrect, whether due to the client unknowingly repeating wrong information, or purposely misleading or minimizing the characteristics of drugs when describing them to the therapist. Regardless, listening to the client should always be a vital source of information for helping that person face the challenges of recovery. When it comes to pharmacology, this goal may be served by the therapist and the client educating each other.

3

Incorporating Art Therapy into Substance Abuse Treatment Programming

The impact of managed care reimbursement systems on SAT delivery has been to mandate use of approaches that are supported by research. These may be referred to as evidence-based, outcomes-based, or best practices. Art therapy may be seen as a welcome alternative approach that enhances, but does not replace, standard treatment approaches. The first part of this chapter looks at the most-used models of SAT and suggests a few ways art therapy can be incorporated; additional suggestions are provided throughout the book. The last part of this chapter includes a case example to exemplify the use of art therapy in individual sessions.

An overview of substance abuse treatment approaches

Alcoholics Anonymous and the Twelve Steps model

Since AA came on the scene in the 1930s, it has been acknowledged as an effective treatment for alcohol problems for millions of people worldwide (Stevens and Smith 2013; White 2014). Its Twelve Steps and self-help group model has been borrowed by fellowships including Narcotics Anonymous (NA) (for users of drugs other than alcohol), Cocaine Anonymous, Overeaters Anonymous, Sex Addicts Anonymous, and many others, which are known generically as Twelve Steps groups.

The variables that appear to make twelve step programs effective also make them difficult to research or to accurately replicate in clinical settings—being strictly self-help, anonymous, and spiritually focused. Although a national office oversees the administrative support of groups through regional bodies and publishes relevant material, AA groups themselves are stand-alone, self-help fellowships, with no clinically trained staff. Group session moderators are chosen from within the group. Closed meetings, arguably the most effective, are open only to those who identify as an addict relevant to that Twelve Steps group. (Open meetings are also open to the public, students, clinicians, and court-mandated people or other potential members who are not willing to identify as addicts.) Members attend meetings only when desired. Progress is measured informally by self-report of time abstinent and by working steps that are grounded in unquantifiable spiritual principles. Participants are never identified beyond their first names during meetings; anonymity is not just a practice, it is a foundational principle that is rigorously defended.

The Minnesota model

Once the gold standard for freestanding SAT programs, this model incorporates Twelve Steps programming with psychoeducation. Original programs made use of recovering counselors and self-help principles. The original model also involved a four-week residential program with an educational curriculum and therapy scheduled throughout each day, which is no longer supported by current reimbursement systems. However, current versions of the model still incorporate twelve step groups (by hosting meetings or recommending that clients attend them in the community) and step work. Some treatment programs require clients to process written worksheets to address the first few steps. The Twelve Steps are covered in more depth in Chapter 7.

Psychoeducation

Psychoeducational groups are a foundation of SAT. It is important for clients to understand the changes in the brain that impact decision-making, behaviors, and cravings; the developmental processes of addiction and recovery; and the impact of addiction on personal and social development. It is generally acknowledged that a person's psychosocial development stalls at the point where the person's life becomes centered round acquiring and using the drugs. It is important to learn and practice mature means of communication, affect regulation, and other social and emotional skills. Psychoeducation is a nonshaming approach to conveying this information and encouraging the development of new skills.

Cognitive Behavioral Therapy (CBT)

Whether they are labeled as such or not, CBT techniques are incorporated into most SAT programs. Practices such as identifying negative self-talk, challenging cognitive distortions, identifying triggers for undesired behaviors, and envisioning alternative coping strategies are commonly employed. Other principles of CBT include teaching clients to handle emotions, problem-solve, communicate effectively, and identify and replace problematic internal self-talk that may be at the root of depression and substance abuse. Rational Emotive Behavior Therapy (REBT) is a frequently used approach for handling emotions, and is discussed further in Chapter 6.

Locus of control

A primary goal of CBT in drug treatment is to balance the client's locus of control or attribution of power over personal circumstances and consequences. Generally, the internal locus of control needs to be strengthened, although counselors of the dominant white American culture should be aware that other cultures may not value individual determinism as highly, or may experience externally imposed limitations that are not encountered by the dominant culture. Among those who abuse substances to the point of presenting for treatment, the internal locus of control is likely to be unhelpfully low, regardless of cultural identity. People with a strong internal locus of control are able to take responsibility for negative outcomes when appropriate, and identify what they can change to avert a future occurrence. They take credit for both successes and failures, believing themselves to be the primary determinants of personal events.

Conversely, a person with an external locus of control may blame others, luck, fate, or other circumstances beyond their control when negative personal events occur. Again, those with disadvantaged statuses or circumstances (or whose addictions are advanced) may be realistic in their perceptions that they have little control over certain life situations. For example, those living in crime-ridden neighborhoods may indeed face greater challenges in maintaining sobriety than can readily be understood by those who have not lived in such situations. Therapists should be ready to inquire about their clients' life circumstances, to assess together the difference between true barriers and evading responsibility, and to assess how personal effort might be invested to improve circumstances.

The Abstinence Violation Effect (AVE) (Barry and Petry 2009) is a concept that relates to locus of control. It refers to the response of a person who has stopped using and then lapses. If the slip is attributed to personal, stable, and global reasons, the person is more likely to fall back into full problematic use. For example, if the self-talk is that "I'm just not that strong a person, and they say heroin is really hard to quit," the person is less likely to recover than if the response is "I was undergoing unusual stress because of that situation at work, but I can get back on track without using again." The importance of self-talk needs to be emphasized throughout the treatment continuum by exploring and personalizing concepts such as the AVE.

Art therapy and Cognitive Behavioral Therapy

Although the pairing of art therapy with CBT may not be immediately logical, prominent writers in the literature (including Matto 1997 and Rosal 2016, first published 1987) have discussed how they are, in fact, a good fit. The process of art making naturally requires considerable cognitive activity, such as uncovering and evaluating mental images, tolerating ambiguity, making decisions, responding to unforeseen events, identifying problems, and generating and implementing solutions. When art products are complete, they continue to be useful for evaluation and the generation of revised ideas or new plans. In a sense, the art making and cognitive processing are in a constant flow of stimulus and response.

Rosal (2016) postulated that art therapists may not be drawn to CBT perspectives because they do not perceive CBT as having to do with emotions, but that it is difficult to separate feelings and thoughts *in vivo*. Both are cognitive processes that drive behavior. Feeling-state drawings can facilitate control over unpleasant feelings or moods by exploring them in an externalized state. In other words, negative feelings can be projected into the art, reducing cognitive distortions, restoring perspective to the client's personal worldview, and making way for increased internal locus of control.

Matto (1997) used the behavioral technique of exposure in art therapy for feelings work by having clients depict their least-troublesome emotions and gradually building up to the depiction of their most threatening ones. The case of Martha, featured later in this chapter, involved elements of these approaches to feelings work in individual art therapy.

Motivational Interviewing and the Stages of Change (MI/SOC)

Researchers DiClemente and Prochaska identified the SOC based on their observations of the way clients navigate the process of personal behavior change (see Connors *et al.* 2013). The researchers sought to use their findings to create a comprehensive, integrative biopsychosocial (BPS) model for behavior change that would be useful for a wide range of populations and settings. The Transtheoretical Model (TTM), casually called SOC, was identified in the early 1980s and has expanded over the years to incorporate a full body of research, theory, and technique. The TTM, together with MI, changed the direction of SAT by suggesting counselors align with clients to enable change processes, rather than confronting and dictating immediate change.

A treatment approach that is applicable to any population, MI is credited to clinical psychologists Miller and Rollnick (2013, first published 1991). It was originally developed in the early 1980s, at about the same time as the SOC. Although the SOC and MI were conceived independently, their authors have done some collaborative publishing, and the two models are frequently used together. MI seeks first to identify the client's conceptualization of the problem behavior and readiness to change. The therapist responds with questions and comments designed to open the client to the possibility of movement along the change continuum. MI techniques are most obviously useful in an initial assessment interview and in the first three stages of the SOC, but are also employed successfully within individual and group counseling modalities throughout the treatment and change process; the therapist's stance is said to employ "the spirit of MI."

This refers to an attitude of respect, compassion, and alignment with the client's perceptions (Miller and Rollnick 2013).

MI and the SOC are effective to help both users and providers of treatment services to conceptualize and normalize the change process. The idea of change as a natural process allows the benefits of a developmental concept, which focuses on assisting the client's individual progress toward a goal, rather than seeking to apply a universal cure for a pathological condition. As with other developmental models, people may at times regress; the stages are not necessarily completed in order, all the way through, or on the first try. The stages are described below (adapted from Connors *et al.* 2013).

Precontemplation

In this stage, the person doesn't recognize use as problematic and has no intention of changing. In the traditional view, a person with a diagnosable SUD and this mindset toward change was characterized as resistant, and the approach was confrontive. Within the SOC conceptualization, such people may be seen as truly in denial, unaware of the consequences or severity of their addiction. In some cases, the person may have attempted to quit but failed, and is hopeless about trying again. Liberal application of the MI approach is recommended when therapists encounter such clients, which is generally only in legally mandated situations.

Contemplation

People in this stage have recognized the need for change, but tend to view the pros and cons of changing as roughly equal. Ambivalence is the hallmark of this stage; those not engaged in a treatment process may remain in this stage for years or even for life. The MI approach features helpful tools for addressing ambivalence.

Preparation

Those in this stage have taken an action toward change within the past year, such as doing an online search for treatment centers or buying a self-help book, and intend to start making the change within a month. When such a person seeks treatment, it is essential to quickly find a placement, although unfortunately, waiting lists are common. It is often possible for people who are in earlier stages to be boosted into this stage if they have been mandated into treatment.

Action
People in this stage have become abstinent and are engaged in making overt modifications to their lifestyle, whether they are in a treatment program, using a self-help group, or working on their own. Relapse is a clear and present danger, and the focus is on defining, individualizing, and working a daily program of recovery.

Maintenance
The maintenance phase is characterized by increased confidence in the ability to stay sober, comfort with a recovery identity, and a declining reliance on special tools or activities to avoid slips. However, the possibility of relapse is still present to varying degrees, so that relapse prevention awareness is maintained and tactics employed when needed. This phase may last for anywhere from six months to five years or more into sobriety.

Termination
This stage is characterized by the person no longer experiencing a temptation to use, no matter how anxious, stressed, or angry they become, or whatever the occasion. They are considered to have 100 percent self-sufficiency; their lives and behaviors are not discernible from those of abstinent people without an addiction history. (This is not to be confused with a cure—the person is not able to return to substance use.) Not everyone reaches this stage; for some, ongoing "maintenance" is a worthy goal or achievement.

Historical support for Motivational Interviewing/Stages of Change-type philosophies in addiction treatment
It is important for therapists new to the addiction field to understand some of the history of treatment approaches, for they may encounter agencies or colleagues whose approach is still grounded in earlier attitudes, which can vary widely. MI/SOC approaches have roots in thoughts espoused by early peer alcohol counselors and AA sponsors that "you have to meet 'em where they're at." But in the 1960s–1980s, the newly emerging field of formal addiction treatment was likely to view resistance and denial as stubborn wrong-headedness, and to apply a one-size-fits-all treatment geared toward a prototypical white, middle- to upper-class, male alcoholic with grandiose behaviors. This stereotyped idea of a client was viewed

as needing to be taken down a notch, and in some residential settings, behavioral tactics included having clients wear diapers for being a narcissistic baby, or a toilet seat around the neck for being "on the pity pot." It is now understood that many so-called treatment failures were not people inherently incapable of recovery as supposed; they simply did not respond well to the confrontational, shaming approach.

Along with the perceived need for confrontation was a common belief that an addict had to "hit bottom" in order for treatment to work. "Bottom" was defined as a point of despair or vulnerability when enough consequences had accrued that the addict was no longer able to maintain denial of an addiction problem. Father Joseph Martin, an early populist alcohol treatment trainer, made an important point about this kind of thinking. Father Martin recalled the proverb, "You can lead a horse to water, but you can't make him drink," which appears to support the conventional wisdom about waiting to treat until someone hits bottom. However, he added a twist: "but you *can* make him thirsty" (Martin 1972). Treatment providers can't force clients to change, but they can educate them and make change attractive.

The concept of "attraction, not promotion" has been one of AA's philosophies since its inception (AA 2001, first published 1939). This concept reappears in the MI and SOC philosophies, for example, in the MI technique for addressing ambivalence that is known as *developing discrepancies*. Therapists use this technique to help the client articulate the difference between a client's current life situation and their goals or values, eventually assisting the client to acknowledge the behavior that prohibits goal attainment.

MI echoes the humanist tradition in that the therapist holds a belief in everyone's ability to evolve into a healthier person. The role of the therapist is to respectfully help identify roadblocks to change. Elicitation of *change talk* is an essential MI tool that builds on the premise that attitudes are changed by speech: people become more committed to what they hear themselves saying. They must be led to speak for themselves, however, rather than parroting the counselor. Art therapists can encourage variants on verbal change talk with art products.

Being human, a counselor is prone to respond in a reactive manner when the solution to a person's problem is utterly obvious, but the person insists on speaking around the issue. It takes mindfulness and skill to refrain from lecturing and instead to ask questions or make comments that lead clients to their own discovery of the situation or solution. By engaging a client with art activities of their choosing, the mindful art therapist supports client control of the session, while seeking openings to elicit change talk, identify discrepancies, and help resolve ambivalence. The MI approach is more difficult for the therapist than the old-school confrontational approach, but it is also invigorating and rewarding.

Developing discrepancies with Josie

Josie was a single mother in her early 20s with a four-year-old daughter, Emma, who would be joining her soon at the women's residential treatment center. Irresponsible behaviors resulting from her drinking had led to several consequences for Josie: a citation for driving under the influence, loss of her job as a nurse assistant, and her caring but concerned stepmother's intention to seek legal custody of Emma if Josie did not stop drinking. Josie had agreed to participate in this particular treatment program because it allowed women to have their children under the age of 12 with them. However, the intake assessment indicated that Josie's motivation to maintain sobriety for the long term seemed questionable. In an art therapy session, we were able to *develop discrepancies* in a powerful way.

On the day of her first art therapy session, I sought to align with Josie by doing a conjoint scribble and asking about her experience in art making. Josie said she used to love to draw and make crafts as a child, but hadn't done so for quite some time. I identified this as a strength and asked her to tell me more about it. Her face began to shine as she explained that Emma's fifth birthday was approaching, and she wondered if she could use the agency art materials to make her a birthday card. She proceeded to choose stickers, markers, colored paper, and glitter glue pens to make an appealing card. This activity both delighted and saddened Josie as she seemed to connect with some deeper feelings about her daughter that had been minimized or denied, probably due to shame over her problems with alcohol. She was showing emotion and engagement for the first time at the treatment center. This glimpse of heartfelt motive regarding her daughter provided fodder for gentle exploration of the discrepancy between continued alcohol use and its probable impact on her ability to be the kind of mother she wished to be for her child. The need for abstinence in her case had already been supported by what she had learned in psychoeducational groups.

Josie's growth through the treatment process began with this session. Developing the discrepancy between her goal of being a good mother and wishfully thinking she could also drink allowed her to overcome remaining ambivalence toward sobriety. Josie was supported in an ongoing manner through phases and stages of change. In a group art therapy session close to her successful discharge, she created a bridge drawing depicting herself and her child departing from her former life into a challenging environment (see Figure 3.1). However, she has heavily emphasized the reinforcements of the bridge, representing community self-help and other recovery tools; her movement toward the future, her child in tow, is depicted as sure and determined.

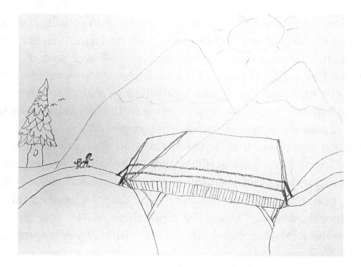

Figure 3.1: Josie's mountain bridge

Individual modality

Yalom (2009, first published 2002) recommended that therapists "create a new therapy for each patient" which is implemented upon the foundation of a trusting therapeutic relationship (p.34). When art therapists fall into the rut of repeatedly using the same preplanned directives with their individual clients, they may not be seeing their distinct needs. In addition, they are missing out on the opportunity to co-create the evolution of the treatment by engaging the client in topics and tasks that arise spontaneously.

These thoughts are of particular importance for art therapists who may be unfamiliar with the addiction population and who therefore may tend to view these clients as a homogeneous group. It is helpful to engage the client in an initial assessment, even if someone else in the agency has already performed a standard intake. This is the opportunity to see how the client presents to you as the art therapist, and to start to build the relationship on a more personal note. Even after the first session, it is important to observe the client's presentation and spoken issues when they arrive for the appointment, rather than automatically applying a preplanned art directive.

A consensus panel of researchers and clinical experts in the addictions field that was convened by a US federal agency recommended several strategies for addiction counselors. Many of the tasks reflect the MI/SOC philosophy, including an individualized, strengths-based focus that does not homogenize the population; a therapeutic relationship that uses respect and empathy rather than authority; a view of treatment as evolutionary and responsive; and incorporation of a variety of approaches to address the needs of the whole person (CSAT 1999). The latter phrase in particular seems to open the door for art therapy. Group therapy provides clear benefits for this population, but due to the tight structure of many treatment curriculums that require group sessions, individual treatment may provide the best opportunity to provide individualized motivational enhancement and create an evolutionary treatment plan using art therapy.

Rhoda's wine bag

I worked with one woman individually who was a multidrug user and valued the sensory and perceptual qualities of being high. She found she could experience similar pleasure by making art, such as colorful paintings in an optical (op) art style, mosaic-like magazine collages, and wall hangings compiled from random pieces of colorful discarded fabric, buttons, ribbons, and natural materials. In the piece shown in Figure 3.2, she transformed a fabric wine bag by hanging it upside down in a symbolic act of pouring out or letting go; she then devised a means of hanging the piece (a support system), using natural, wholesome materials; and finally, she decorated it (that is, awarded the changed object or self) with buttons, like strings of medals. The piece and the symbols evolved together in a pleasing and recovery-affirming experience. Although to an outside observer we were simply making crafts, I was able to articulate the project and its metaphors for change as movement toward goals in her treatment record.

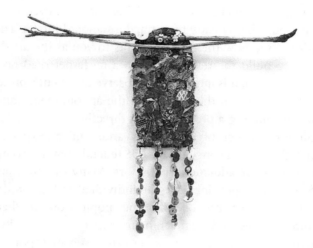

Figure 3.2: Rhoda's transformed wine bag (see color plate)

The case of Martha

The treatment plan for Martha, a client in a residential program, included the use of cognitive behavioral art therapy to do feelings work by *in vivo* exposure, as well as to employ cognitive mapping for recovery planning. Drawing assessment tasks were used to gain insight; understandings of her drawings and of her ego defenses were partly informed by psychodynamic theory. For the most part, I kept my interpretations to myself; we focused on Martha's ideas about her own drawings. The therapeutic approach was humanistic and incorporated techniques of MI. Martha liked to draw and was a volunteer for individual art therapy sessions; she also attended my art therapy group as well as the mandated agency groups and individual sessions. I was able to see her for only three individual art therapy sessions, but I believe they made a significant difference in the quality and outcome of her treatment, as well as in her level of engagement with the other aspects of treatment.

Profile

Martha was a 37-year-old woman on probation for a second offense of drug possession. She was mandated to drug treatment by her probation officer after having tested positive for cocaine (in her case, crack) twice in the past month during routine drug screens. Martha indicated at her intake that she was tired of her addiction and the problems it had caused, and was ready to change.

After her first criminal offense, Martha had attended outpatient treatment and managed to remain sober for almost a year. She attributed her relapse to stress over being unemployed, having to live with her mother, and difficulty regaining her 15-year-old son's trust in her. Prior to becoming dependent on crack, Martha had worked for eight years as a teacher's aide in a preschool, a job that she loved, and had lived independently with her son. Her son's father now lived in another state and was not involved with the family; he had been verbally and emotionally abusive to Martha. Martha had never known her own father. Her mother had long-term sobriety from an alcohol use disorder and was condemnatory toward Martha regarding her addiction. Martha's son had responded to her irregular parenting by turning to Martha's mother and sister, which added to Martha's low self-esteem and shame. As she was to realize in treatment, when Martha's usual defenses of intellectualization and isolation of affect failed to suppress her painful feelings, she sought the blissful oblivion of a crack high.

As I formulated her individual art therapy treatment goals, I buttressed the goals she had set with her agency counselor: relapse prevention planning, learning to access her feelings, and learning communication skills to improve family dynamics. I realized that her characterization of her relapse trigger as "stress" was somewhat generic and defensive, and that shame and even self-hatred were probably closer to the mark. In addition, she seemed to have some unmet narcissistic needs from having had an absent father and a mother who had had her own relationship wounds and addiction, and who was now righteous and cold in her recovery. Notwithstanding her family-of-origin issues, it was apparent from our initial conversation that Martha had, in her earlier adulthood, been a confident and capable person who had been blindsided by the biological juggernaut of crack cocaine relatively late in life. Her shame was not difficult to understand.

Session 1: Goals and assessment

My intention for this session was to get to know Martha better and administer baseline drawing tasks, including a drawing and memory screen for organicity, a Kinetic Family Drawing (K-F-D), and a Kinetic House-Tree-Person (K-H-T-P) drawing. Martha was at ease in the individual setting; her eye contact was direct without being challenging. She often commented or chatted as she drew. She came close to expressing upset feelings relating to an instance when her son had gone to her sister for advice; she seemed hurt that he had not come to her, but also seemed to quickly shrug off the feeling before it could really register.

I told Martha that it was great that she could identify situations where she had probably experienced uncomfortable feelings around her relationship with her son. Then I asked whether she preferred not to really feel her feelings, and how that might play into relapse for her. Obviously, this was not the first time she had come across this concept, but the art tasks provided a new angle for exploring the topic. She agreed that art making might be a good way to get in touch with her feelings, thereby reducing the emotional factor in the vicious cycle of her drug abuse. I suggested that we might also use a task to help her understand their relationship from her son's point of view, which would enable better communication with him in the future.

Art impressions

In Martha's K-F-D (see Figure 3.3), she and her son are seated across the long ends of the table from each other, which might suggest emotional distance. The mother serves as the go-between, both logistically in the picture and in real life. Both of her mother's hands are placed firmly on the tabletop in an attitude of control. Although Martha described the image as her family having fun playing a card game, she herself seems to be turning to leave her chair, perhaps symbolizing that she felt less included in this prosaic family scene, or perhaps more broadly reflecting her discomfort and avowed need to get out into her own house again.

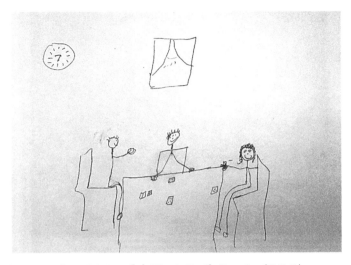

Figure 3.3: Martha's Kinetic Family Drawing (K-F-D)

The inclusion of the clock seemed to indicate an awareness of the passage of time. When I asked about it, Martha responded concretely that they had a clock on that wall. Then almost immediately she referenced time in a distressed manner, saying it was going by so fast and that she did not have many years left to live with her son before he would be on his own.

The immature graphic style of the K-F-D may reflect Martha's own sense of being immature at age 37, living with her mother, and having her mother provide for her son. It may also reflect a reluctance to dwell on an emotionally provocative issue, that of her family relations. Martha's mother is a constant reminder of someone who was successful after the first try at abstinence. Although Martha depicts herself with a smile in the K-F-D, her aspect is almost that of a naughty child about to sneak off from the dinner table before being excused.

After seeing this drawing, I asked Martha to try not to make stick figures, and she complied readily. When she made the K-H-T-P drawing (see Figure 3.4), Martha appeared more confident and to enjoy the drawing experience more; she commented cheerily about the apples and flowers as she added them. This make-believe subject matter was much less threatening than her family, and the happy content is reminiscent of her use of defenses such as isolation of affect and reaction formation.

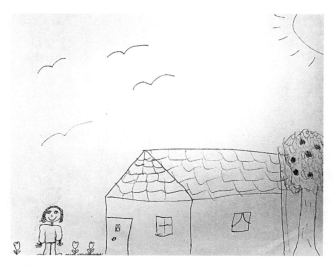

Figure 3.4: Martha's Kinetic House-Tree-Person (K-H-T-P) drawing

Session 2: Goals and assessment

Just before the session started, another counselor briefed me about a situation that had developed the previous evening after most staff had left. One of the clients had managed to get some drugs smuggled into the facility, which had caused an uproar, and resulted in several people relapsing and one being discharged. In her role as the client liaison, a position assigned weekly to a deserving resident, Martha had acted appropriately to try to resolve issues among residents and report to staff as the drama evolved.

Although my original plan had not included any kind of check-in drawing, I decided to have Martha do a reaction drawing to this event; I was hopeful that it would call up some emotions for her.

I also wanted to proceed with my plan to have Martha use oil pastels to create an abstract-feelings drawing. Although in some instances abstract drawing might serve to enable *distance* from emotions, I believed that Martha's intellectualization and rationalization were enabled by her concrete symbolic and representational drawings. I would also be bumping her out of her media comfort zone of pencils or fine-tipped marker pens. After processing this piece, we would discuss her termination and post-treatment plans, and if time allowed, I would ask her to make a drawing about going home.

Martha seemed impatient when discussing the previous day's chaos. She seemed exasperated that people couldn't resist temptation, even in this relatively safe treatment setting. As in other instances when her tone, increased speed of speech, and other indicators of emotionality began to emerge, Martha quickly shut herself down by saying "Oh well, that's just how *that* is." At the same time, as Martha moved closer to treatment completion, I had observed that she seemed to be more willing to explore feelings like anxiety, especially with regard to starting over in recovery. Threats to sobriety were expressed vividly in her work from art therapy group that week, which involved a stream-of-consciousness written response to an image of a person going over a waterfall in a barrel, as well as in a crazed flame-headed symbol of addiction in her incident drawing, which she firmly isolated by enclosing it in a thick green boundary.

Art impression

For the abstract-feelings task, Martha produced a color-saturated red and black motif for anger and fear, perseverating on it for a short while in a seeming attempt to define and master it, saying, "It's like when your anger and fear are all mixed together, and then the other person's anger and fear get mixed in too." She said she had been talking with her primary addictions counselor about how her family's avoidance of any kind of unpleasantness had, in fact, led to fear of what others were thinking or feeling, along with frustration, repressed anger, and resentment. In her motif for shame, a small teal-colored self/circle seemed smothered and suspended within a black box set in a corner of the paper—the same location as the box depicting home in her K-H-T-P and other drawings. When I observed her body language and facial expression, Martha appeared to have accessed deeper feelings during this session, but remained tied to intellectualized verbal descriptions.

When we moved on to a going-home piece, which was meant to help her relax after doing the more unpleasant feelings work, Martha quickly connected with a feeling almost of bliss as she seems to float home to her child (see Figure 3.5). Martha sometimes used an odd schema for drawing bodies that could be suggestive of a cognitive confusion or sexual trauma. When I asked about her unique schema, she explained proudly that she had developed the way of drawing a person with a circle and two curving lines, and always thought it was cool. In this going-home drawing, Martha used a marker stamp of musical notes scattered in the sky above her to emphasize her happiness at the homecoming. The expression on her face as she drew this piece and the fond tone in her voice when describing it imbued this drawing with sincerity; however, it also represents denial, a dreamy escape. When her drawings were independent of dominant associations to home or her son, such as in her cognitive mapping task and incident drawing, Martha seemed more competent and grounded in reality. By comparison, the images that featured home also featured anxiety, fantasy, or both.

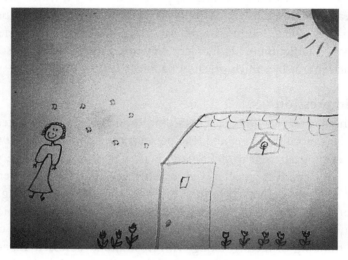

Figure 3.5: Martha's drawing of going home

Session 3: Goals and assessment

I had observed that Martha seemed to think of her son in an almost stereotypical manner, as though she did not really know him as an individual. I attributed this to the fact that her eight-year addiction had derailed her attention to him as he was growing from a young boy into his own person as an adolescent. A more empathetic knowledge of his viewpoint might improve their relationship, the deterioration of which was a major relapse trigger. The agenda for our final individual art therapy session was as follows:

1. Make a cognitive map drawing to express concepts and plans for a new life in recovery; process verbally to reveal strengths and possible red flags.

2. Make a free drawing with oil pastels to explore the feelings her son has toward her, as a means of desensitization, and to serve as a basis of empathy on which she can practice newly learned communication skills.

3. Compare the first and last drawings made during treatment to identify and solidify gains and facilitate closure.

Art impression

The graphic cognitive mapping task, which involved structure and creating symbols for triggers and safe activities, was predictably appealing to Martha. Although she included two stick people (one in a representation of herself dancing through the rest of her "probadtion"—a misspelled label I silently enjoyed as a Freudian slip), these were symbolic shortcuts. The repetition of money symbols, which were also present in one of Martha's earlier drawings, seemed worthy of note. We discussed the way money was featured in Martha's positive recovery plans to get a job and rent an apartment, as well as in representations of relapse triggers, as when she had "extra cash lying around." When I enquired, Martha stated she did not have or know how to open a bank account, so I spent a few minutes addressing this necessity for her successful recovery. People in early recovery, particularly someone Martha's age, often feel embarrassed that they have never performed basic life tasks such as this, and may avoid asking for help. I was glad to see that Martha's primary depiction of herself in this drawing was firmly grounded, with squared shoulders, and on a clear path to the front door of a tall building labeled NA (Narcotics Anonymous) that looked nothing like her home/shame box schema.

In the second drawing of the session, which explored her son's feelings toward her, Martha's self image appeared totally regressed (see Figure 3.6); this seemed to underscore her successful affective connection with her subject matter. Her body was drawn with an even more bizarre version of her usual odd schema, which may reveal the shame and ego disintegration she felt on receipt of the overwhelming emotions being relayed from her son's much larger figure. Her arms now resemble breasts, symbols of mother-nurturing that in her case has been rejected. The long, sketchy necks—an attempt to separate the cognitive head from the anxiety-producing emotional body—appear to echo her need to avoid the acknowledgement of painful emotional states. In corresponding affective confusion, her face simultaneously portrays a half-smile and tears. In the emotional experiencing of her angry and betrayed son, Martha appeared to have felt powerless, and regressed to a distorted recreation of her childhood schema.

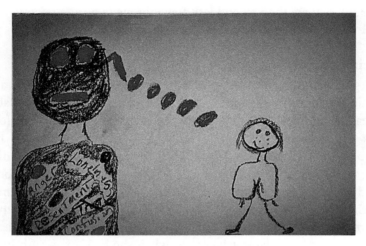

Figure 3.6: Martha and her son's feelings toward her (see color plate)

Several motifs were repeated from the previous session's abstract-feelings drawing, including the use of colored dots to depict emotions residing in a black box, in this case one that became her son's body. This time, she labeled the dots, perhaps in an attempt to catalog these feelings of her son's. His black head with red eyes and other red marks was reminiscent of the black and red motif she made to depict the combination of anger and fear that she had processed in last week's drawing.

As this drawing progressed, Martha displayed increasing signs of distress such as sighing, frowning, pressing her lips together, and adjusting her chair. The red line connecting her son to herself was added last, as she explained, "He never really *says* what he's feeling; he just gives me *that look*." Then, as she began describing the drawing further, tears formed in her eyes and she allowed them to fall without wiping them away.

After we were able to verbally discuss her tearful response, we looked at the very first drawing Martha made in treatment, which had been in art therapy group (see Figure 3.7). The directive was for clients to draw or depict something about themselves, using representational drawing or symbols; they were allowed to write words if desired. Martha had made a very concrete, decorative piece featuring colorful hearts and her own and her son's first names (in the figure, pseudonyms were written in her style and placed over the original). The piece had the naïve look of one done by an adolescent girl about her first boyfriend; when she had shared it in group, Martha had talked about her son as if they hadn't a care in the world. Her previous denial of reality couldn't have become more apparent after the experience of this session. Again, Martha's tears fell. I told her that I didn't doubt that love existed between her and her son. By comparing the pictures, I wasn't trying to say, that is what you used to think, and what you made today is the only reality. She said she understood, and even verbalized some of the metaphor. Before, she had been totally unable or unwilling to own any of the negative emotions connected with their relationship; she had been, as she put it, "hiding behind the happy hearts." Now she was capable of making a very powerful picture of another part of their relationship, and of experiencing emotions instead of avoiding them. By learning how to do this, she was making it possible to have a real, and really loving, relationship with her son.

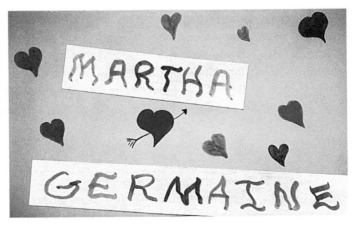

Figure 3.7: Martha's first drawing, "Happy hearts"

This final session provided the hoped-for successful finish to our brief course of art therapy. Martha was able to experience her negative feelings, to acknowledge them verbally, and to allow me to see the evidence of their existence, and to observe that the world did not end when this occurred. After crying, she stated that she did not like feeling her emotions to that extent, but that it was not so bad after all, and definitely not worth going back to the "crack craziness."

Martha was able to consolidate lessons from various aspects of her treatment experience. She told me that in several treatment modalities, including art therapy, she had been helped to understand that a great part of her family's dysfunction was due to anxiety surrounding the expression of emotions. Appropriate modeling of negative emotions did not occur during her upbringing: anger and fear could not be displayed, which confirmed the covert message of their dreadful power. Her mother had modeled dealing with any discomfort, internal or external, by drinking, and after her recovery, by rigid suppression. Also, both women had experienced relationships with men that had been emotionally abusive. This seemed to intensify the competition to bring up Martha's son as each saw fit, which involved infantilization by Martha, and an overemphasis on control by her mother.

Martha had come to realize that the understanding she had gained about the etiological factors contributing to her drug abuse was helpful, but just a beginning. She reflected with a wry smile that becoming sober only set you up for further work. Martha acknowledged that for her, this meant continuing to practice tolerating her own feelings, becoming aware of and correcting cognitive distortions, and learning to model and receive an appropriate expression of feeling when communicating with her son. When I suggested that she ask her son to draw with her sometime, she seemed sincerely taken with this idea. Having just proven to herself the power of art to communicate, she was ready to add this new tool to others she had acquired in treatment.

Summary

This case exemplifies how art therapy can quickly access emotion and lead to insight. Martha experienced and expressed emotional pain in the final session, and realized it was tolerable, and not worth "going through the crack craziness" to avoid feelings in the future. Her progress in accepting her feelings over just three weeks' time was powerfully revealed by comparing her first and last drawings.

Martha developed a conscious understanding of the need to feel and express her emotions, both to stop her personal pattern of addictive behavior, and to create genuine relationships with her son and other family members. Martha realized she liked to draw and could continue to make drawings to access feelings and order her thoughts. She thought that drawing helped her become aware when she was starting to use intellectualization and similar defenses to cover up feelings, and to take this as a warning sign that she was entering a cycle of emotional avoidance that usually ended in relapse. She could also invite her son to join her in drawing for fun. Martha had learned by drawing with me that this is a way to triangulate pressure in a two-way relationship and to make talking easier.

Martha favored defenses such as intellectualization and isolation of affect rather than more provocative ones like displacement or acting out, which contributed to genial therapeutic relationships with staff. She reacted to questions, comments, or suggestions without becoming defensive, as so many substance abuse clients do. At the same time, her tendency to remain on an intellectual plane precluded deeper emotional processing. While she appeared to be a leader in groups, in actuality she was also hiding. The use of art therapy in individual sessions made the difference in Martha's ability to break through defenses regarding her feelings and relationships. Without it, her progress and prognosis would have been much less positive.

Conclusion: factors in success

No single approach guarantees success in SAT, whether it is the Twelve Steps, MI/SOC, pharmacotherapy, or art therapy. Similarly, each individual's case contains many variables that will contribute to or stymie progress. In the case of Rhoda described above, who was self-referred to my private practice, we had the luxury of extended session time in the studio as well as treatment time that extended over many months. She had the financial resources to stock her home with a range of art, craft, and fiber tools and supplies, and the avid creative drive to spend time making things just for the joy of it.

When working with the two other women represented in this chapter, I believed I built therapeutic relationships that were as strong as could be managed in just a few sessions, and applied principles of art therapy that were individualized to each client's needs. I believed that in both cases, the art therapy provided a significant turning point, enabling greater success in the overall treatment episode. Yet I was also highly aware of other factors that were perhaps just as essential to their overall success, which are summarized in Table 3.1. Awareness of these types of holistic factors can inform therapist and agency planning and decisions.

Table 3.1 Analyzing positive outcomes for Josie and Martha

Factors category	Specific factors in Josie's success	Specific factors in Martha's success
The treatment system	Availability of a setting that allowed her to have her child with her and that offered parenting classes and support	Legal system referral that interrupted her addicted "life as usual" and mandated the choice between treatment and prison
Client protective factors	Job training; devotion to daughter; past enjoyment of creative hobbies; likely support of stepmother if sobriety was achieved	Relatively older; solid former work history; prior success in recovery and positive experience of sober lifestyle; sober friends and family
Personal strengths shown by the client in treatment	Ability to tolerate enough vulnerability to build therapeutic relationships with therapists	Interest in drawing and art therapy and willingness to take the risk to use art to work on the goal of accessing feelings
The art therapy	Flexibility to allow the client to make a sticker card rather than the art therapist requiring adherence to a planned agenda or insisting on a more artistic directive	Experimentation with both abstract and pictographic depictions, using both graphite and more sensory media, to access emotion and facilitate cognitive processes
Characteristics of the art therapist	Nonshaming style in an authority figure, where the client expected judgment	Role of partner and witness in the investigation of feelings, and coach for cognitive mapping
Serendipitous opportunities, capitalized upon in art therapy	Daughter's upcoming birthday prompted desire to make a card; ensuing tender feelings supported developing discrepancies	Other clients' dramatic relapse incident created opportunity to elicit response art and change talk, solidifying commitment to recovery

4

Assessment

This chapter provides an overview of assessment in the field of addiction treatment, the ways in which art therapy assessment can identify client needs, and corresponding treatment goals and interventions. Many drawing tasks are helpful both as assessment tools and as therapeutic applications. Specifics such as commonly found symbols and themes are explored by reviewing the literature and providing case examples.

Substance use assessment and diagnosis

Accurate diagnosis of a SUD and assessment of individual needs, both at intake and as client care evolves, are the foundation for treatment and intervention plans. Research has informed the development of multidimensional assessment rubrics to evaluate the whole person and to determine the best type of treatment; perhaps the most widely used is that developed by the American Society of Addiction Medicine (ASAM 2016). Use of the ASAM criteria is mandatory to enable clients to receive services in most states through US government-funded providers. The criteria assess needs in six dimensions, including detoxification, readiness for change, and home environment. Assessment measures such as the Addiction Severity Index (ASI) and Substance Abuse Subtle Screening Inventory (SASSI) may be employed at intake to help identify needs in these dimensions and to inform establishment of a treatment plan. Addiction professionals are mandated by a national code of ethics to use "only those assessment instruments whose validity and reliability have been established for the population" (NAADAC 2016, p.12).

In the US, diagnosis of SUD according to the *Diagnostic and Statistical Manual of Mental Disorders* (DSM) is usually a prerequisite for third-party payment for services. The current edition, DSM-5, provides a severity continuum from mild to moderate to severe; the location on this continuum is a major consideration in recommended level of care (APA 2013). The DSM provides separate diagnoses for 11 chemical categories of drugs, but the criteria for each are virtually identical, requiring evidence of "a problematic pattern of [the substance] use leading to clinically significant impairment or distress…occurring within a 12-month period" (APA 2013, p.490). Most of the drug diagnostic categories list 11 symptoms, of which a minimum of two is required for diagnosis; the number of symptoms identified determines the severity specifier for the diagnosis.

Contributions of informal art assessment

Once a diagnosis has been established by formally sanctioned tools, information supplied by art therapists is more likely to be of service. Continued observations and comparisons of client art from early assessment throughout a treatment episode are valuable indicators of client needs and progress. In some instances, art products may signal a need for reevaluation. After inpatient clients have completed detoxification, their presentation may differ significantly; outpatient clients may not be sober or sufficiently detoxed when they are assessed. Forrest (1975) discussed a case where she realized through serial observations of the artwork that a client had a psychotic disorder that was initially masked by alcohol symptomology. Rubin (2011, first published 1984) has pointed out the value of art in teasing out differential diagnoses.

When I worked as an art therapist in a treatment center, I found that the counseling staff welcomed my suggestions for possible changes to the treatment plan based on information I had gleaned from processing informal assessments and other art with the clients. One benefit of art therapy assessment was of particular interest to my addiction counselor colleagues. Many research-supported diagnostic assessments rely upon the honesty of a client's self-reported drug-using behavior. Some clients will lie about whether they use certain drugs or minimize the extent of their use. Others, often younger clients, may "fake bad" to defensively project a tough image, although this is more likely to be done in a group of peers than during an assessment. Art-based assessments, particularly those without a directive that references drugs or addiction, may bypass these types of dishonesty to some degree. Although information gleaned from such evaluations must still be evaluated carefully, they may point to the need for further exploration with the client.

This is not to say that art products produced in drug treatment spring spontaneously from clients' subconscious without passing through a conscious filter. Especially in this very guarded population, drawings may be created to meet the perception of the therapist's preferred response or for social acceptability in a group. In discussing the value of the Bird's Nest Drawing (BND), Kaiser and Deaver (2009) noted that it did not provoke these typical difficulties. This would be true of a task such as the BND, whose metaphor is more obscure to the layperson, than of a task such as the bridge or road drawings, whose projective symbolism is more evident to a person in SAT.

Certainly, unguarded information is more likely to come forth when the client is less aware of metaphorical meaning. Clients whose brains are still befuddled from withdrawal, or who were originally or have become more rigid thinkers, are less likely to perceive potential interpretative themes and are thus less likely to be guarded in choosing content. Therapeutic gains seem most likely when the client becomes aware of the metaphor as they conclude the drawing and are looking it back over. I have witnessed clients experiencing an unexpected insight when they are nearly completed with an art task and suddenly understand what it is revealing about them. The next response can vary, from trying to erase or throw away the drawing, to an excited acceptance of the information and willingness to share it.

Research on drawing assessment related to addiction

Prominent art therapy research related to assessment or diagnosis of people with addiction issues (PWAI) was mentioned in Chapter 1: Francis *et al.* (2003) found that those with SUD were more likely than those not diagnosed with addiction to reveal insecure attachment and to use less color in the BND; and Rockwell and Dunham (2006) found that three of the Formal Elements Art Therapy Scales (FEATS), Realism, Developmental, and Person, correlated to a diagnosis of SUD.

Other studies have sought to correlate features in assessment drawings to features associated with substance use or abuse.

McLachlan and Head (1974) examined human figure drawings of 80 people diagnosed with chronic alcoholism. They identified five characteristics of the drawings that were positively related to previously validated measures of organic brain damage: figure off balance, major detail missing, gross body distortions, weak synthesis, and poor motor control.

Milne and Greenway (2001) measured adults' preferred ego defense styles and sought to correlate them to features of their drawings. Research results were mixed, but a few conclusions were supported regarding defenses commonly used by the substance-abusing population. Passive-aggressiveness and devaluation correlated positively with making dotted patterns. Projection correlated positively with drawing complete people and negatively with drawing patterns; Milne and Greenway theorized that drawing a person allowed for more cathartic experience of projection. This was evidenced in their sample by the preponderance of people drawn in an unattractive, comic style, with small heads or large noses. I have noted use of a similar comic style in free drawings, often with derogatory labeling, in what I interpreted as a defensive manner. The unattractiveness of the people thus drawn (e.g., with crossed eyes, sprouting hairs, tongues sticking out) seems to mirror the inadequacy of the self-image, which finds release in projection.

Common themes and symbols

Cartooning, doodling, and graffiti-style art productions are commonly encountered in SAT. Drug imagery may seem ubiquitous in early stage artwork, particularly with adolescents and with marijuana devotees who have become expert at drawing the familiar palmate leaf; gradually this content fades as the client's world literally enlarges to include other schemas.

Growth may be reflected in art products in an idiosyncratic manner. Some clients' drawing style becomes less chaotic and more structured as they improve during treatment, reflecting increased groundedness and self-control. Alternatively, defensive patterning and rigidity may be replaced with more flexible or emotive articulations. A freer style may become cathartic as the client accesses previously repressed feelings.

Content and symbolism of art productions may also have idiosyncratic interpretations. Knowledge of symbol meanings is helpful for the therapist, not to interpret client art, but to inform further investigation in tandem with the client. It should be explained to clients that there is no one certain meaning behind any art object or symbol in a particular work, and that the art therapist does not have diagnostic superpowers derived from symbol interpretation. Symbols might have universal or archetypal meaning, but they may also have individual meaning based on personal history, or cultural meaning derived from a particular ethnic group or other cultural subpopulation, such as illicit drug users. Even a consciously developed personal symbol may be perceived in a different way if it is revisited at a later time. When the art therapist represents the exploration of the art as an exciting process of discovery, most clients are readily engaged in finding meaning in their work. Some PWAI often think too concretely to volunteer interpretations of their symbols, but I have found that when an array of possibilities is offered, they often become intrigued.

Split faces

Split-face or split-head drawings may not be common, but in my experience they appeared regularly enough to be notable. In Luzzatto's (1987) research that asked people in SAT ($n=50$) to depict their self/internal world and object/external world in a single drawing, 20 percent of the participants further split the self into good and bad halves. The split-self motif may reflect the dualism or splitting that characterizes the self-perceptions, or perhaps more accurately, self-deceptions, of people with addictions. This splitting differs from the dissociative splitting that occurs with sexual trauma patients; while I have observed the latter depicting themselves as dual whole figures, this is a different presentation than the face or head divided vertically in half I have observed with clients in SAT. Of course, many have experienced both trauma and substance abuse issues. Heidi's split-head art product is discussed in Chapter 6.

The stigma, shame, and guilt incurred by abusing substances are imperfectly defended against by further abusing substances. Splitting is another means of psychic defense. Unable to integrate the good and bad aspects of themselves, some clients seem to befriend the split, or even to glorify it; they may brag about having a dual nature, like Dr Jekyll and Mr Hyde. Others describe a feeling of alienation or helplessness that their original good self has been stolen or possessed.

Still others appear to be aware of a split, but are ambivalent or unmoved by it. A client who presents a relatively harmonized split-face drawing may not yet be aware of the need for change, or is unwilling to admit it. Richard's drawing was suggested by a prompt to draw the sober self and the using self; it was his decision to combine the two in one face (see Figure 4.1).

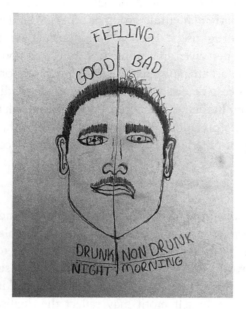

Figure 4.1: Richard's split-face drawing

The sameness between the two halves is apparent. The expression on both sides is bland, although the mouth is turned up on the Feeling Good/Drunk/Night side, and down on the Feeling Bad/Non-drunk/Morning side. He described the fried-looking hair treatment on the right side as "when you're so hung over even your hair hurts." Richard's drawing reveals his defensiveness about his habit and ambivalence toward recovery.

Marquette was a teen I worked with individually in my private practice who was abusing a variety of drugs. Marquette was bright and inquisitive; we had previously discussed the adolescent search for identity, and how drug abuse could figure in to that dynamic in a normal way, but also become a problem. Early in treatment, Marquette created the split-face drawing in Figure 4.2 as a response to my request to "depict a mask you wear;" I had suggested this theme because I had intuitively questioned his sexual orientation or gender identity and hoped to provide an opportunity for him to be forthcoming. The resulting drawing was more explicit than I had hoped or anticipated. Marquette's split mask appears masculine, and half covers a feminine-looking face. The somewhat feminine colorway of the male side's sweater was representative of Marquette's personal style of dress. While he was working on the drawing, Marquette chatted in a blatantly casual manner about people he knew who were gay, bisexual, and transgender; he was testing my tolerance for diversity. When he had finished, he grabbed a marker, added the title with a defensive flourish, and then declined to discuss the drawing or topic further. However, the image was so arresting and its message seemed so clear, it did not seem unreasonable for me to bring it out from his file in a later session for a "portfolio review." Thus, after many sessions, Marquette got up the courage to tell me that he believed he was meant to be a female. This in turn allowed me to connect him to supportive groups in the community that would also support his goals for recovery.

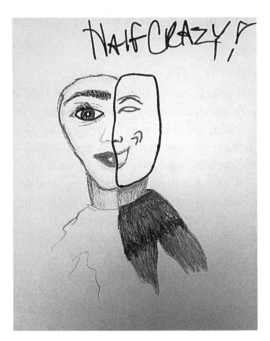

Figure 4.2: Marquette's half mask (see color plate)

Formal and informal projective assessment
Limitations and alternatives to traditional projective drawings

Analysis of content in projective drawings can produce misleading labels, and is not supported for diagnostic purposes (Groth-Marnat and Wright 2016). Raters may unknowingly project personal material or values, or interpret content based on theoretical preferences or preconceived expectations of the client. Art therapy measures such as rating systems of the Formal Elements Art Therapy Scale (FEATS) and the Diagnostic Drawing Series (DDS), which focus on formal drawing elements or structures rather than on content, show promise as diagnostic tools. At this time, research is ongoing and work specifically involving addiction diagnoses has been limited (Mills 2015). Use of the Expressive Therapies Continuum (ETC) as an informal assessment and treatment planning tool has been well articulated by Hinz (2009a, 2009b). Clients can be assessed for their developmental operating level in various situations. Although use of the FEATS, DDS, ETC, and various drawing tasks do not serve formal diagnostic purposes, they can provide a deeper insight into the nature of a client's addiction and suggest direction for therapeutic interventions or further assessment.

Interpretation

Formal projective assessment as described in the field of psychology has tended to focus on pathology by equating elements of the drawing with pathological symptoms. In the earlier days of projective assessment, oral fixation and narcissism were more entrenched in definitions of alcoholism, and this theory found application in the interpretation of drawing content. For example, the disproportionately large person, mouth, and eyes in one K-H-T-P drawing earned a case study label of "Alcoholic Hedonist" (Burns 1987, p.38). Arguably, there is assessment value in such diagnostic snapshots, but if allowed into the therapeutic relationship, this kind of labeling would only stereotype and disrespect the client (even were that label updated to "Person with alcohol use disorder who prioritizes pleasure-seeking"!).

For art therapists, the ultimate value of assessment is to guide therapy, and the most beneficial assessment is done with an awareness of strengths-based and developmental approaches. Other means of avoiding a pathological focus (or interpretative projection) are to observe the client making the art, involve the client in a discussion of the art, use a variety of client drawings rather than only one for assessment purposes, and include free drawings in the assessment collection. These approaches also lessen the likelihood that the client produces work designed to please the therapist.

Interpreter projection: Jerry's bridge drawing

Professionals working in SAT become accustomed to hearing stories of past trauma and reading client histories filled with adverse childhood experiences. While it is essential to hold these likelihoods in mind when looking at client drawings, it is also important to guard both against assuming them, and against the tendency to project negative meaning from the overall feeling given by a drawing. In actuality, the client may be responding literally to a prompt and the drawing may have a relatively benign or idiosyncratic meaning. Figure 4.3 shows a bridge drawing made during an art therapy group in response to the prompt, *draw a picture that has a bridge and a person in it. You may add anything else you like.* I had not yet met Jerry, the client who produced this drawing; he was attending this drop-in art therapy group as an alternative to a recreational activity at the treatment center. My immediate unspoken interpretation of his drawing was that he felt inadequate, helpless, and hopeless. I discounted the smile as a ubiquitous example of reaction formation, and projected myself into what I perceived as a woebegone, childlike self figure. I felt the despair of being stuck under a railway bridge, with no escape route in sight, and an ominous certainty that a train would roar overhead at any moment and cause the flimsy structure to collapse on my ill-fated Charlie Brown head.

I received a reality check when volunteers in the group shared about their bridge drawings and stories, and Jerry chatted happily about a childhood memory of playing hide and seek under an unused bridge over a dried-up riverbed on his grandparents' farm. Of course, I could still ponder, "But why did *this* image appear? Why now? Is there a deeper meaning?" I did not have the opportunity to pursue those questions with Jerry, but I did relearn an important lesson about double-checking my overwrought assumptions!

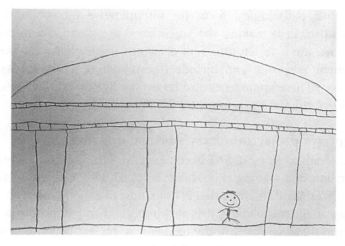

Figure 4.3: Jerry's bridge drawing

Media

Another factor to consider when applying projective assessment is that although this population is frequently described as creative, when faced with a drawing task that appears to be a test of realistic drawing ability, many clients will be uncomfortable. Free drawings may provide richer, more valuable content for guiding therapeutic interventions and reassessing goals. However, clients may be equally threatened by nonstructured drawing tasks. Providing a choice of media often eases these difficulties, and some clients are better able to express themselves with painting or dimensional media than with drawing utensils. Graphic development researcher Golomb (2004, first published 1992) observed that if participants were allowed to choose the art media with which to complete a developmental assessment task, scores improved. The art therapist's observation of a client's choice of media provides input for assessment and indicates best options for future therapeutic interventions.

Red flags

Formal elements or content in the drawing that seem to identify pathology or hidden concerns, sometimes referred to as *red flags*, may be the therapist's projections. Therapists who are new in the profession or unfamiliar with the subculture of addiction may overreact to what is a norm for the population; for example, they may respond with exasperation or cynicism when an adolescent spends his first hour in art therapy drawing a beautifully detailed marijuana leaf. To put this in perspective, the therapist might think about how a person who is highly committed to athletics would be likely to doodle or make free drawings featuring balls, scoreboards, or other items relevant to their sport. Many people immersed in the drug culture draw paraphernalia and drugs; I believe the first level of interpretation should be a simple awareness that this is a normal human response. Unfortunately, some treatment settings, often those for adolescents or in corrections, prohibit such drawing. Although the rationale for this is certainly arguable, it is more helpful, within individual art therapy sessions and especially in the beginning, to allow freedom for clients to express themselves in whatever way is most comfortable.

The treatment center philosophy may rightly see such images as glorification of the drug or culture, and they do not want to promote that; however, these drawings may also represent an ego-defensive stance that is more about repeating forms that are reassuring to make and contemplate. Art therapists over the years have recommended that such imagery be accepted in noncritical fashion and that clients not be moved away too quickly from activities that support defenses. Hinz (2009b) expressed this concept within the framework of the ETC when she wrote that excessive functioning within the perceptual level of the ETC is indicated in the repetition of stereotyped imagery. She recommended beginning at the level where the client is naturally comfortable, looking for any deviation in the artwork that indicates movement toward a higher level of the continuum, and encouraging expansion in that direction.

Prognostication: hindsight is 20/20

It has been noted in the literature that drawings made in treatment settings may feature prodromes or have prognostic value, although sometimes this is realized only in retrospect. Several bridge and K-H-T-P drawings I have gathered over the years were, in hindsight, quite predictive of relapse or of dropping out of treatment. Some of these drawings included the three indicators named by Dickman *et al.* (1996) as potentially predictive of relapse (drugs or paraphernalia, lack of articulated figure, and geometric style), but so did the drawings of many other clients who did not drop out or relapse.

In my experience, instances of prognostication are anecdotal, but fascinating. At times, clients literally paint a picture of their intentions regarding treatment; these drawings often have an "in your face" quality that suggest an authority-challenging motivation (Schmanke 2016). Occasionally I have wondered whether such drawings were done in full consciousness, or whether they might be a covert cry for help. Clients who actually draw themselves in the process of using drugs may fall into this ambiguous category; to draw this type of action is notably more intense than simply depicting the favorite drug. Depicting other types of regressive actions may also suggest a turning away from recovery.

Sondra drew herself in a small boat beneath a sprawling traffic bridge, rowing furiously to the left (avoiding future consequences) toward a tropical island (see Figure 4.4). She explained that the person was going to "take a vacation instead of taking the bridge to work." Sondra actually absconded from residential treatment during the night after making this drawing. Her roommate told staff that Sondra's boyfriend, a drug smuggler, had arranged to have a plane ticket to Florida dropped over the fence at an assigned spot, and off she went, leaving the hard work of the treatment bridge behind.

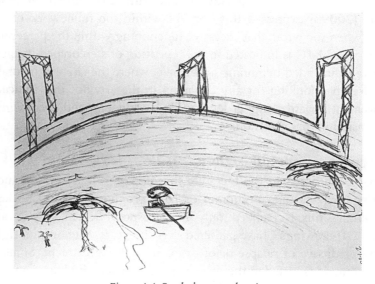

Figure 4.4: Sondra's escape drawing

Metaphorical and projective drawing tasks

Despite pitfalls if used in a traditional manner, psychological projective drawing tasks used for informal assessment with this population can be informative and therapeutic. The K-H-T-P drawing (Burns 1987) is often the first drawing I request. Its innocuous subject matter tends to be reassuring to clients, who frequently comment about lack of drawing skill rather than becoming defensive about potential interpretations. The K-F-D (Burns and Kaufman 1972), or an animal version, which may be less threatening and more revealing, provides an insight into family of origin or current family dynamics. Etiological factors and needs for adjustment in family functioning in order to support recovery are readily identified. Asking a client to Draw a Person in the Rain (DAPR) (Hammer 1958) can provide a snapshot of a client's perceptions of stress load and personal capability.

Drawing assessments developed by art therapists that have been described with the substance abuse population include the bridge drawing (Hays and Lyons 1981), road drawing (Hanes 1995), Bird's Nest Drawing (BND) (Kaiser 1996), and the amusement park technique (Hrenko and Willis 1996). Other examples of tasks that can inform assessment and therapeutic interventions with this population include the incident drawing (Cox and Price 1990) and crisis directive (Holt and Kaiser 2009).

As affirmed in MI/SOC approaches, assessing a client's own identification of their problem is an important foundation for directing treatment planning. Themes for several popular drawings involve picturing the client's problem or problematic situation. Cox and Price (1990) asked adolescents in SAT to *draw about an incident that occurred during the time you were drinking/drugging*. They discussed the therapeutic benefits of these drawings, particularly when shared in group: they help break down denial, allow participants to express feelings, and explore values and alternative behaviors. Holt and Kaiser (2009) created the First Step Series to generate change talk using creative directives within an MI framework. The first activity, the crisis directive (*draw the crisis or event that brought you here*), assists in the evaluation of the client's perception of the problem and readiness to seek help. Directing clients simply to *draw your problem* is my favorite approach. The ensuing depiction of content can assist in evaluating a client's perspective and sense of responsibility. For instance, do they draw their drug of choice, themselves, an unhappy family situation, a legal authority, or a jail cell (Schmanke 2006)?

Haluzan (2012) identified factors associated with personal competence when she asked clients with addiction issues to *draw yourself in a positive environment*, and noted that a majority of figures appeared to be disoriented or lacking in initiative, and often seemed to be far from home, such as in the mountains or a forest. She related this to difficulty functioning in complex situations, the search for a place of one's own, and feeling more comfortable in isolation from relationships. Wadeson (2010) described three art directives to assess aspects of familial alcoholism. These involved asking the individuals to make symbolic depictions of the family; make symbolic depictions of the two grandparent families; and depict the influence of alcohol consumption on the family. She was stuck by the concordance of symbol choice among family members, when they had not seen each other's drawings until all were finished.

Road drawings

Asking clients to draw a road comes off as a relatively nonthreatening request, but results may be deeply symbolic when clients, whether consciously or not, depict the path of their drug addiction. Hanes (1995) described universal elements of the road metaphor, and also warned against overlooking idiosyncratic meaning. In reviewing the road drawing of a client with a heroin addiction, he noted that the client consciously used stereotypical symbols of his addiction, such as a sign reading "Dead End;" further analysis with the client led to insight from idiosyncratic symbols such as a heart-shaped syringe.

Draw a Person in the Rain (DAPR)

DAPR is a projective task that was first discussed in print by psychologist Emanuel Hammer (1958). He described several clinical examples, usually comparing his clients' Draw a Person (DAP) images with their DAPRs, and finding that indicators of pathology tended to be hidden in the former but would emerge in the latter. Hammer's case illustrations included a convicted criminal whose DAP figure was bluff and manly, whereas the one in his DAPR was puny and worried-looking; Hammer described the patient's original compensatory persona crumbling under stress.

Verinis, Lichtenberg, and Henrich (1974) found that a broad diagnostic category (neurotic, character disorder, or psychotic/borderline) could be predicted at a better-than-chance rate by assessment of DAPRs with no further information. Willis, Joy, and Kaiser (2010) studied DAPRs of 40 people diagnosed with co-occurring disorders, and identified a trend toward significant positive correlation between protective features in the drawings (such as outerwear, an open umbrella, an item in the environment providing shelter) and scores on a coping-resources measure.

Used informally, the DAPR is suggestive of two factors: the client's perception of current environmental stress, and the client's perception of their own coping resources. The addiction population frequently reveals a high level of perceived environmental stress. This stress level may be at its height during the time of intake; most clients' lives are in chaos, and they have been externally pressured to go to treatment, whether via family, school, employers, physicians, or the legal system. I have observed many drawings (not necessarily DAPRs) that depict the client directly beneath a dark cloud that is raining down only on them. The presence or absence of protective features (which include indicators such as the person smiling or dancing in the rain) further inform interpretation and may be suggestive of the direction of the client's locus of control.

The amusement park technique

In developing the amusement park technique with inpatient dual diagnosis groups, Hrenko and Willis (1996) found it elicited discussions of powerlessness and similar themes associated with substance abuse. They noted that the directive to *draw an amusement park event, ride, or booth that represents your life* seemed fun and invited patient participation; in addition, it provided assessment information for the therapist. Hrenko and Willis identified correlations between the experiences of the amusement park rides and the experience of substance use or addiction, including highs and lows, repeating cycles, loss of control, overstimulation, risk-taking, and danger.

In a family assessment session, Barry depicted his newly formed family riding a roller coaster in an amusement park drawing (see Figure 4.5). Barry's wife was in recovery and successfully involved in a twelve step program; his first wife, and mother of the family's two children, was actively abusing substances. Current stressors included custody and boundary issues; in addition, Barry's children were moving through puberty and evincing dramatic, although developmentally normal, behaviors of their own. Barry described the roller coaster as "fun, something we all like to do together, but it's also scary, because you can't always see what's coming up around the bend." When he was queried about the prominent low building he had depicted beneath the family on the ride, he shrugged it off, saying he was trying to make an accurate depiction of the local theme park. Then he quickly exclaimed, "You know, it's like maintenance. That's me!" He had correctly identified one of his important roles, as a dependable support for his family's heady new structure.

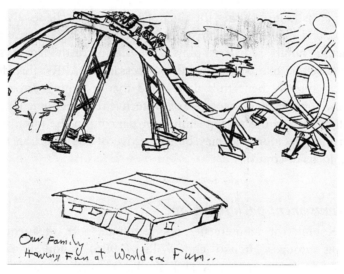

Figure 4.5: Barry's amusement park drawing

Bridge drawings

Hays and Lyons (1981) noted the many symbolic connotations of bridges when developing their seminal bridge drawing: they are a means of communication or connection, a way to solve problems or overcome obstacles on one's path, signs of achievement and progress, and transitions to a better place. They explored their directive with a nonclinical adolescent population ($n=150$), and also described it as a treatment tool with patients in SAT. Those populations were seen as being "in transition" or a state of major personal change, and therefore more likely to respond subconsciously to the bridge metaphor. The authors identified 12 variables of interest in the drawings, which included the solidity of the bridge, the nature of the matter under the bridge, and the location and direction of movement of the self in the picture. They noted that in Western cultures at least, movement from left to right signifies positive movement toward the future. In addition to using drawings from these populations to research the task, they processed the drawings in treatment groups with the substance abuse population, and found it to be effective both as an informal projective assessment and as a prompt for interpersonal feedback in groups.

The Hays and Lyons directive requests clients to *draw a picture of a bridge going from someplace to someplace.* When most are done, they are asked to put a dot in the picture where "you" are, and an arrow to indicate the direction of travel (1981, p.208). Holt and Kaiser (2009) varied the prompt for their recovery bridge drawing, instructing clients to "Complete a bridge depicting where you have been, where you are now, and where you want to be in relation to your recovery" (p.247).

When I began to use the bridge drawing in SAT, I wanted the additional assessment value of having clients draw a person. In addition, I thought the projective nature of the task was one of its primary values, so I avoided in the directions any explanation of the bridge as a recovery or other metaphor. My prompt has been *draw a picture that has a bridge and a person in it. You can add anything else you want.* Table 4.1 shows a matrix I developed to guide informal assessment with the client or discussion in a group. I have also explored variables of interest in addition to the 12 identified by Hays and Lyons, to include paper spanning, use of vertical orientation, and use of words on the drawing.

Table 4.1 Elements of the bridge-drawing task (Schmanke version*)

	Obstacle (usually water)	Bridge	Environment—left of bridge	Environment—right of bridge	Person
Metaphorical meaning	The thing that blocks the developmental life path	The aid to getting beyond the obstacle	Life situation that is no longer viable/acceptable	Life aspiration necessary to wholeness or actualization	Self/the one on the life journey
Symbolic of	Addiction and consequences	Tools or assistance in recovery (treatment)	Life as addict (may include life leading up to addiction)	Life in recovery/happier, healthier life	Self/client
Temporal location	Past, present, or just recent	Present	Past	Future	According to placement in drawing
Possible red flags for assessment/discussion points during treatment	Inviting, distracting, hypnotic; threatening, especially if bridge is precarious	Precarious, unstable, ineffectual, paper-sided; overly detailed or sketchy	Attractive, bland, or similar to right side	Extravagant, overly trite, or similar to left side	Placement off bridge; features indicating incompetence, ambiguity, or despair

* This table provides suggestions to enable therapeutic use of the bridge drawing, using the prompt, *draw a picture that has a bridge and a person in it. You can add anything else you want.*

Paper spanning

In 2004, I examined variables in over 70 sets of bridge drawings and stories by people in SAT (Schmanke 2005). In tallying particular drawing features within this collection, the most noteworthy finding was the great number of drawings wherein the bridge spanned the entire page, with no environment on either side. Because I omitted the references to places on either side of the bridge in my version of the directions (although I do suggest that they can add anything else in addition to the person and bridge), paper spanning was obviously more likely to occur than if I had used Hays and Lyons' directive with its reference to a bridge going *from someplace to someplace* or Holt and Kaiser's more complex direction.

As I looked closer, I realized that this appeared to be related to the type of treatment the client was in: the bridge spanned the page in 63 percent of the drawings by residential clients, but did so in only 32 percent of drawings by participants in outpatient settings. I surmised that this reflected the inpatients' more intense immersion in the treatment (bridge) experience. Looking further into the data, I noted a trend that among outpatients, those who completed treatment successfully did not make bridges that spanned the page, whereas those who later dropped out were more likely to have made paper-spanning bridges. This finding might be interpreted to support the importance of the proper placement setting to client success.

Vertical orientation

Another finding of interest was that very few clients, about 7 percent of my sample, chose to use the paper in a vertical position. My procedure was to set out materials for groups in advance, either on a separate table or counter, or randomly set in the middle of smaller round group tables. Thus, the paper was not placed in any particular orientation in front of the clients prior to drawing. Hays and Lyons reported that 84 percent of their initial adolescent group chose a horizontal placement; they pointed out that a bridge does suggest a horizontal positioning. They further speculated that the narrower vertical placement would discourage placement of material at either side of the bridge, and thus perhaps served as a defense against making connections with the bridge.

It has been observed elsewhere in the literature that "Horizontal drawings tend to tell a story and vertical drawings tend to make a statement" (Furth 2002, p.35). To imagine a person and a bridge insinuates the process of crossing a bridge, which requires motion through time and space; this does relate to the telling of a story and the need for left-to-right room on the page. The vertical drawings in my collection offered plausible anecdotal evidence for the concept of vertical drawings making a statement, or, as I thought of it, a *snapshot*, compared to the horizontal's *video*, and they also affirmed Hays and Lyons' view of the vertical as defensive.

Labeling

Another variable, that of writing or labeling directly on the drawing, seemed also to be indicative of defensiveness. Although writing on the drawing was found in only 3 of the 66 horizontally oriented drawings (Al's bridge, discussed in Chapter 8, was one of these), it was found in three of the five vertical drawings, and seemed to affirm their defensive quality. Labeling or explaining something in words is a left-brained or analytic activity, compared to revealing a concept or story in images; it may be more prone to involve mental censorship or deceit. Use of words on drawings may reflect a need for the client to avoid or deny emerging material and relabel it as something else, or it may indicate a desire to steer the therapist into a certain interpretation.

In one of the labeled vertical drawings, the person crossing the bridge is literally making a statement in an attempt to impress me, his counselor (see Figure 4.6). Lon had written in a cartoon speech bubble coming from his stick-person head: "Hey Libby I'm going to a [NA] meeting." The bridge is paper-sided, and the person is not moving forward toward the future meeting, but is standing facing the viewer. Two huge clouds fill the sky above the person's head. These features may unconsciously represent the two powerful authorities that Lon needed to appease to stay out of prison: the substance abuse agency and the community corrections program. But the tilt of the bridge and its precipitous slant to the left/past suggests that the poorly outfitted/equipped person, despite his cheery smile and reassuring words, might rather readily slip or fall back into using and dealing.

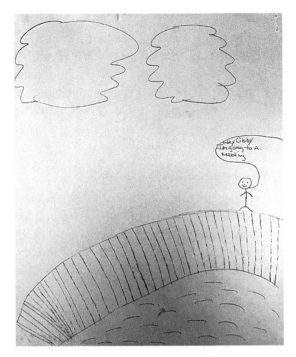

Figure 4.6: Lon's vertical bridge drawing

Another labeled vertical bridge drawing in the collection depicted a popular electronic game that featured stacked layers of challenging environments including a river and a traffic bridge. I interpreted the implicit statement presented here as, "I am going to play the game, and attempt to win my way through treatment, but without revealing any of my true story." The written bridge stories for both these vertical drawings were predictable, reflecting the overt content of the drawings. In general, most of the clients' bridge stories were mundane and uninteresting, even when covert meaning boiled out of the corresponding drawing. Such is the ability of the defenses to prevail when words are used, whereas unintended revelations often slip through in art products.

The bridge drawing is effective for a variety of uses, and I am continually amazed at the variety of presentations it elicits. By giving the directive in a manner that does not reveal the metaphor, it is helpful for initial informal assessment. When used as a therapeutic intervention, particularly in a group session, the bridge drawing prompts helpful interactions among group members, who are usually quick to perceive the metaphor during the discussion stage if they have not done so already while drawing. Feedback from a group is more readily accepted by the artist, who is confronted with his own art production as proof when defensive or other problematic patterns are unveiled (Schmanke 2016). Even after the metaphor of the bridge is fully realized, the task can be revisited over time to address the client's current stage of change.

Conclusion

Art products are likely to reveal information otherwise withheld by a population that tends to be taciturn about its problem behaviors for a variety of reasons. Of course, no drawing should be used in isolation to form conclusions about a client. Allowance should always be made for idiosyncratic meaning. The client's explanation of the art is important collateral information, and although a verbal or written explanation may appear to be contradictory, this is in itself a helpful indication of a defense. Clients who are too defended or rigidly concrete-minded to explore symbolic meaning may soften after experiencing such exploration by others in a group. The therapist and client may glean insights in individual sessions by revisiting earlier drawings together as treatment progresses. Assessment of client art can inform initial evaluations, and perhaps more importantly, feed the evolution of treatment plans and agendas.

5

Group Work

Group work is foundational in SAT. Some program designs include both smaller interactive therapy groups and larger psychoeducational or lecture-style groups. In others, especially in smaller agencies, these are combined. Many programs require clients to attend self-help meetings while still in treatment; they may be encouraged to identify a meeting that they feel comfortable with to become their *home group* after discharge. (Information about self-help groups is given in Chapters 3, 7, 9 and Appendix B.) Aftercare or continuing-care models often involve groups.

This chapter examines the benefits of groups and group art therapy, models of group art therapy, special issues for substance abuse groups, and considerations for group stages, including group identity on the Stages of Change continuum. The literature review on this topic from Chapter 1 is supplemented to provide more detail. Case vignettes and sample activities are included; see Appendix A for additional suggestions for group directives.

Benefits of group work

Benefits of group work for this population include a reduction in the sense of isolation, shame, and internalized stigma; observation of successful peer recovery; and interpersonal feedback, which is more readily accepted from peers than from the therapist (CSAT 2005). Yalom's research (with Leszcz 2005, first published Yalom 1970) identified 11 therapeutic factors of group therapy that serve as a foundation for interactive-style groups. Factors that are particularly relevant for SAT include the instillation of hope, universality, cohesiveness, and the creation of a social microcosm in which to work through relational issues. A focus on here-and-now processing keeps these clients from getting bogged down in *war stories* (grandiose recounting of past drug usage or other dramatic experiences).

Group art therapy provides benefits over group verbal therapy, such as offering a less threatening mode of communication and easing the discomfort of being required to participate verbally in group. Art therapist Riley (2001) explored how the addition of imagery to group therapy intensifies therapeutic factors like universality and interpersonal learning, and helps to keep group process in the here-and-now. Art making in a group setting allows introverted members to be more expressive, while talkative ones can be silenced during the image creation (Waller 1993). Riley advocated for therapists to acknowledge any effort at the activity without judgment or correction; particularly for clients new to the group, any mark, stick figure, use of written words, etc. was accepted. This approach aligns with the spirit of Motivational Interviewing (MI), which requires the therapist to meet the client where they are, instead of insisting on meeting a higher goal at the onset of treatment. Another art therapy principle espoused by Riley and others that supports the MI spirit of respect is to disallow interpretations of the art unless by the art maker.

Modeling and teaching respect is especially important when working with the substance-abusing population, which tends to have its own cultural hierarchy (mothers of young children are usually the pariahs). Facilitators need to be cognizant of their own feelings in order to create a group culture where no one shames another. Winship (1999) noted that people in SAT typically don't want to be close to others in an unguarded way out of fear of rejection, yet, when initial resistance is overcome, real work is readily accomplished. The resultant cohesiveness is healing in itself, as well as serving as a support for further work. Even the understanding and internalization of psychoeducational material is more robust when a treatment cohort has become cohesive through therapeutic group experiences.

Art therapy group models

It is likely that most group work done by art therapists in SAT will follow an interactive or interpersonal-style verbal model, rather than an analytical-style one. Arts-based or studio models, while effective, may not fit into inflexible curriculums of most managed care treatment settings, and are more likely to be found as an optional offering in a milieu setting.

A commonly used structure for interactive-style art therapy group sessions has been explicated and described by Skaife and Huet (1998) as the *sonata form* for its similarities to that musical construct. The three-part session opens with coming together and identifying a theme; then moves to working individually on various interpretations of the theme through the artwork; finally coming back into group process for verbal revisiting of the theme. This approach works well when provision of art therapy requires adherence to a psychoeducational curriculum. The use of check-in drawings in place of the traditional verbal check-in at the beginning of group can enliven the process as well as encourage a more personalized application of theme material. Skaife and Huet's model also incorporates typical participant concerns for each movement, such as worrying about whether there will be enough time to finish a piece, or whether verbal sharing will be required. The facilitator's awareness of such likely concerns is necessary to make conscious decisions about whether those concerns are to be allayed or allowed to exist as part of the process.

Inpatient and residential treatment are more likely to provide open studio settings as part of a milieu approach. Art therapy in such instances may be seen as an activity therapy or adjunct treatment. An art therapist in such a position may have relative freedom to encourage more personal and in-depth art experiences; a workshop studio setting incorporating an art-as-therapy approach was preferred by Wittenberg (1975) for adolescents in residential SAT. At the same time, in such settings art therapists may not be allowed to read patient files or be able to design individualized treatment protocols.

Group stages and Motivational Interviewing/ Stages of Change approaches

There seems to be general consensus among group theorists that interactive groups proceed along a developmental path that includes:

1. An initial stage, where members observe each other, form impressions, and generate norms.

2. A conflict stage, where members drop their overly cooperative personas or negotiate for control; conflict may ensue

between members, or hostility directed by members toward the therapist.

3. A working stage, wherein the group matures in its identity and behavior, becomes cohesive, and works toward goals, with gradually reduced input from the therapist (Yalom with Leszcz 2005).

A closed group with an unchanging roster is most likely to make textbook progress through distinct stages. However, even groups in open-entry programs, where new clients enter and other clients complete or leave, rarely start over at the first stage whenever enrollment changes. Usually such groups will vacillate within the later stages, depending on personalities and shifts in morale within the group. Therapists working in substance abuse should be prepared for defensive acting out of various kinds to take place in groups, particularly in the conflict stage, but potentially at any time.

Although usually the SOC model is applied to individuals, MI/SOC principles are important considerations in group work as well. When possible, it is helpful to establish groups according to the readiness of the clients for change. This may be done at the initial referral level when, for instance, those in the pre-contemplation stage are referred via the correctional system to a program such as Alcohol Information School, or chronic relapsing clients are referred to settings where active-stage groups work toward establishment of abstinence and relapse prevention.

Screening methods and Stages of Change early-stage groups

Preliminary individual screening is beneficial to ensure a good fit of the client for the group. Even where options do not exist and the client must be placed in a particular group, individual prep can be used to go over group norms and dynamics, ensuring the client's informed entry into an already established group. An individual session also allows for tailoring an introduction to art therapy aspects of the program. Clients can be asked questions such as whether they have experienced art therapy, when the last time was they used art materials, and what kind of experience they had with art or other creative activities growing up.

If time allows in a pre-group session, I like to ask the client to draw a Kinetic House-Tree-Person (K-H-T-P), chosen for its apparently innocuous subject matter and its ability to tell me about the client's drawing ability. When they have finished, I ask them to tell me about it; we may ponder whether it has any particular symbolic meaning, but I do not offer an interpretation. I stress that, despite what they may have seen on TV, art therapists do not go about analyzing people on the basis of a single drawing, and when they are in group, their own verbal interpretation of their work, whatever they may wish to share, will be honored as truth. Particularly if the client still seems confused or disquieted, I may point out something in the drawing that I see as representing a strength, and suggest it to the client as an example of what I mean by processing their work. This must be done honestly, but I have never *not* been able to identify some positive symbol or quality. This serves to depathologize the situation and leave the introductory session on a positive note. I have demonstrated that I can see good in them, and further, that it is not my imagination, but is reflected in the strength they have revealed in their drawing.

In settings with enough numbers and resources, a group prep session for newcomers before they are assigned to therapy groups is another option. Research has indicated that pre-group prep groups featuring MI techniques result in significant improvement in participation over other pre-group approaches (Walitzer, Dermen, and Connors 1999). These techniques include normalizing ambivalence about treatment and developing discrepancies between clients' present behaviors and their desired life situations.

Normalizing ambivalence can also be accomplished through group art tasks. Simple graphic directives can be used to introduce art therapy at a level that doesn't challenge artistic skill and can also serve as icebreakers, allowing group members to share more easily about themselves. For example, they can be asked to *draw a thermometer that shows how cold or warm you are toward treatment* or to *make a simple drawing of the thing that is your primary motivation for being here*. Clients develop a greater sense of interest in each other when from the beginning they see that others in their treatment setting may be at varying stages of readiness for change.

A model for action stage interactive art therapy groups

The group model described below is geared toward clients in the late preparation or action stage, who are no longer struggling with ambivalence. It is a process-type group, rather than a psychoeducational group, although it may involve a psychoeducational or life skill focus. Art activities may be employed at any point to explore confusion, generate solutions, evaluate progress, or celebrate success. A narrative example is provided in the case of Jay.

When new members are rotating in or until a group is well established, open each group with a reminder of group norms (although this use of the term is strictly inaccurate, it is usually better received by the population than *rules*). The content should reassure clients by focusing on respect and safety, and might include guidelines such as these:

- confidentiality is to be observed (most agencies have their own language for this; "what is said in here stays in here" is a popular version)

- members are there to help each other, and discussion should flow between members rather than through the therapist

- the atmosphere should be one of respect and encouragement for all, regardless of diagnosis, drug of choice, stage in treatment, or any other personal characteristic

- members have different art abilities, and all who make an effort to express themselves through art are respected, and

- the group is to be nonconfrontational and nonargumentative, but disagreement may be expressed by personalizing with "I" statements and suggesting a constructive alternative.

In open topic groups, members are asked to share their goals and progress, including any stumbling blocks, and to give encouraging feedback to each other. Therapists should guide processing toward the here-and-now, to avoid exploration of personal history, etiology, or war stories. Usually, the group agrees by consensus to address one volunteer's problem in that session, but it is understood that the process helps all.

As a structure for group sessions, the following action-oriented steps are reviewed:

1. Restate commitment to personal goals.

2. Identify skills needed to change behavior patterns.

3. Problem-solve ways to change or acquire those skills.
4. Test or practice skills by role-playing.
5. Explore possible barriers to change.
6. Identify concrete action steps (homework).
7. Follow up in the next group session by reporting and evaluating success of the action steps.

Art tasks can be interjected at any point where emphasis or clarification is desired. For example, the person may depict his problem as the first picture in a cartoon strip, and group members brainstorm solutions by drawing the end of the strip, or group members can choose magazine collage images to represent skills needed to address the problem. The focal person may interact or respond to these suggestions using art materials as well. Art products can be displayed in the group room if appropriate, or kept and reviewed at appropriate times.

Jay's group: assertiveness role-play with masks

Jay was an openly gay man in his late 20s who said his drinking was out of control. He was in intensive outpatient treatment after his attempts to stay sober on his own had failed. Our treatment model was geared toward action stage participants, and in group sessions, we educated the clients about the Stages of Change (SOC) and enforced a group culture of mutual respect and support. In a sense, we trained members to be co-facilitators; a bulleted list of group principles and techniques, similar to those given above, was posted prominently on the group room wall.

The format for the art therapy group was to explore a theme derived from topics in the psychoeducational group. Group members would volunteer personal issues related to the topic, and by consensus the group would choose one member on whom to focus. We would then brainstorm an art activity that might help. A volunteer from the group performed the role of "scribe" to record the focus client's primary observations during the session. This transcript was included in the client's treatment file, and a copy given to the client as well, which helped reinforce gains when it was read later.

In the session described here, the psychoeducational group topic had been assertiveness skills. The art therapy group supported Jay's desire to develop these skills by staging a puppet role-play to help him practice changes in behavior. Using puppets or masks, rather than directly role-playing, can help clients overcome self-consciousness and try out new behaviors more easily. Additionally, the person who is playing the foil to the client is less likely to be easy on that person or to stop the role-play prematurely.

Jay began the process by sharing his thoughts: "I feel like I am really ready to quit drinking, and I am willing to make changes, but in some areas I feel stuck. I still like the social atmosphere in a bar... I know it's not a good idea to spend time there, but it's harder to find other ways to socialize when you're gay." Rather than taking a confrontational approach (such as accusing Jay of making excuses), the facilitator and group employed the Motivational Interviewing (MI) spirit and praised Jay for his commitment to change. The facilitator asked how he thought improved assertiveness skills could help.

"I think part of why I drank was about not feeling good about myself in relationships. I let people take advantage of me... I would pay their bills and enable their drinking and drugging, then they would just treat me like shit anyway; it's like they lost their respect for me. And really I guess I lost respect for myself too. I need to learn to say no and mean it!" One group member joked that the next time someone approached him wanting something, he should "just say, *fuck no!*" Jay laughed but continued: "Actually, I do need to learn to say no more easily like that when people ask me for favors. I always have the best intentions, but then I'll meet some charming guy..."

One of the experienced group members proposed a mask role-play; another suggested the assertiveness storyboard exercise (see Appendix A). It was decided to incorporate both concepts. Jay was invited to sort through a box of "masks," which were magazine images of people's faces that were fairly close to life size. These had been precut, mounted on cardboard, and attached to a craft stick, so that they could be held in front of the role-player's face. The selection included anonymous people showing various emotions as well as a few celebrities, which often prompted symbolic associations. Jay was directed to choose four faces: one for a passive, one an aggressive, one an assertive version of himself, and one representing his nemesis, "a charming guy asking for a favor." He chose a picture of a handsome popular singer for the latter, and pictures of noncelebrities for himself, including a child holding her hands in front of her face for his passive persona. He was then directed to choose a group member to use the celebrity mask and play the charming nemesis; his choice did a convincing job.

Moments of friendly laughter and approval at the choice of masks, combined with the group's support and his own motivation, enabled Jay to earnestly tackle this role-play. When he had demonstrated his ability to speak passively, aggressively, and finally assertively to his nemesis, he stated, "You know, doing all that just made it seem so obvious that *I have options*. I don't have to be tied down to my usual way of reacting. I can pick a response and *act* like I'm this guy here, put up the Mr Assertive mask, even if it doesn't come naturally right away." As a therapeutic reminder, I took a picture of Jay with his Mr Assertive mask and printed the picture for him to keep along with his copy of the narrative provided by his scribe. (Remember to investigate agency regulations and ethical considerations before photographing clients.)

Another group member respectfully reflected back on the pros and cons of the gay bar issue. He brought up the well-known advice to "change playmates and playgrounds" in sobriety. Hanging out in bars with charming freeloaders was a high-risk situation for Jay, not just because of the availability of alcohol, but because of the greater risk of falling back into unhealthy relationship patterns that served as triggers. To wrap up this discussion, the group helped Jay specify two action steps he was willing to practice and report back to the group in a week. These were "I will be assertive at least once a day by appropriately refusing a minor request; or by asking for something, such as at a restaurant or store; or by speaking up to voice my opinion in a conversation" and "I will not go out to the bar unless I am with a friend who doesn't drink and who knows about my weaknesses and my recovery plan."

Jay felt accomplished and much more optimistic about his ability to change after the supportive experience and structured outcome of this session. As the facilitator, I was sure that the masks had made this a deeper and more productive experience than it would have been if we had used a standard role-play. Even when clients are not producing the art themselves, the function of images for projection, the added layers of symbolic meaning they provide, the increased comfort level of experimenting with roles behind a mask, and the aspects of play and humor are all important values of art therapy in groups.

Special issues in group work
Narcissism and the false self

Art therapist Springham (1998) discussed the pathological narcissism of the substance-abusing population and the likelihood that patients will *appear* to engage in therapy, but often this is from the false self or treatment persona. By comparing information from privately completed questionnaires with disclosures made in group process, he found that the more narcissistically defended the client, the greater the discrepancy between private and public disclosures. By observing others who share appropriately in a cohesive group, clients with narcissistic tendencies may soften their resistance to risk-taking in this regard. Springham also found that this work is positively impacted by *individual* art making in the group setting, which allows for withdrawal into narcissistic reverie before coming back into the verbal group processing phase. At that point, negative transference, repressed grief, and similar material conveyed in the imagery can be processed at a safer distance than through verbal expression alone.

Liebmann (2004) described group art therapy in a hospital alcohol unit in which a more directive approach was used to address the problem of the false self: members were asked to paint the masks they perceived each other wearing. As with many directives that have the potential to shame, the art therapist should consider the maturity and cohesiveness of the group before proceeding, and perhaps set parameters on the verbal processing or responses. While peer feedback often precipitates a breakthrough, treatment may be derailed for someone who feels disrespected in front of the group.

Addiction treatment expert C.C. Nuckols (2016) also believed that breaking through narcissism is essential to lasting recovery, and that group work was the most effective approach, since direction from an authority figure is not likely to be accepted. Instead, group therapists can build a culture where clients who are at a later stage of recovery share "I used to think like you" feedback in a kindly way with the narcissist. Another approach Nuckols described involved the use of imagery to encourage naturally self-centered clients to enlarge their worldview and remain open-minded to new ways of achieving change. In sessions, he used a striking photograph of a Himalayan scene in which tall mountain peaks rise above the shoulders of lesser mountains, in turn rising above foothills. Clients are asked to pretend they are at a particular point partway up, then to close their eyes and imagine, "When you look out, would the world look different to you than it did when you left the foot of the mountain? Now, pretend you're further up…now at the top…will the world seem bigger or different than you imagined? Will you be able to see things you couldn't see before?" The mountaintop self-portrait activity is an effective complement to themes of narcissism, humility, perspective, and achievement (see Appendix A).

Group imagery

Canty (2009) explored the concept of the "key image" that emerged during drug treatment sessions. Such an image, expressed in the art of one member, was found to be a universal theme that spoke for multiple group members. Springham (1998) also explored the concept of the group image; he provided an example of an image identified by a SAT group as a magpie's eye, which revealed negative transference of the group onto the art therapist as a beady-eyed observer. McNeilly (2006) and Skaife and Huet (1998) referred to the psychological concept of "resonance," or unconscious linkage between group members, revealed in the unintentional production of like images in art therapy groups. In the case of resonance and the production of similar imagery, more suspicious clients may perceive that group members are surreptitiously "copying" another's work. The therapist can assure them that while sometimes this may be the case, it is not rare for group members to unknowingly create the same image or symbol; it is almost as if the group is telling itself where to go in order to process important issues. The therapist can guide discussion by asking for emotional responses or brainstorming about meanings. By keeping the tone curious, rigid interpretations are avoided and freer thinking encouraged, which is always of value to this population.

A situation that is similar but psychodynamically different than resonance occurs when more than one group member uses the same stereotypical imagery. The group therapist may tire of seeing rainbows and hearts in depictions of life in recovery. However, it can be interesting to engage group members' thoughts about such imagery. In one adolescent group session, when clients had been asked to make a bridge drawing, Judy and Marissa created drawings featuring similarly styled daisies and tulips (see Figures 5.1 and 5.2). The similarity of the flowers drew the attention of the group, though the girls were not sitting near each other and no one thought either had copied. This similarity was an easy thing for group members to remark upon without anyone feeling threatened. But it was also obvious that while Judy's landscape was the same on both sides of her bridge, Marissa's showed a great contrast. In both, the flowers appeared to represent things going well; in Judy's, the insinuation was that the interruption of treatment (the bridge) in her landscape would not make a difference in her life. Seeming to suddenly perceive that this was obvious to everyone, Judy then announced defiantly that she was in treatment only because her parents had put her there, and that she had no intention of stopping her marijuana use. Sometimes a defensively produced group image provides unexpected grist for the mill: exploring the similarities of these drawings provided an opening to their more revelatory contrasts.

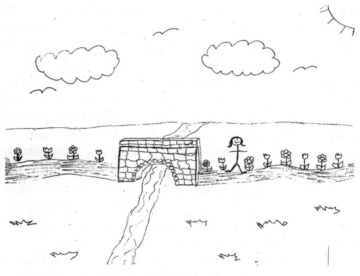

Figure 5.1: Judy's bridge of no change

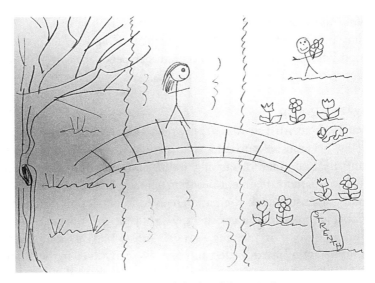

Figure 5.2: Marissa's bridge of dramatic change

The therapist's role

Groups are dynamic systems, and working as a group therapist requires alert observational skills and a more extemporaneous response than individual work. Most treatment programs feature open groups, where service users are admitted and discharged in an ongoing fashion, as opposed to closed groups with stable membership. Dynamics may shift and alliances change as members come and go. Therapists must be mindful to build cohesion, which is best done by encouraging a culture of caring respect, affirming attendance and participation, watching for problematic subgrouping or scapegoating, and allowing the group to have a voice in rules and processing (Yalom with Leszcz 2005). The less authoritative style that is typical of a group facilitator in the interactive model enhances cohesiveness and interpersonal learning. Groups should be discouraged from getting into the rut of verbally sharing by "going around the circle" to process individually with the therapist.

Some clients will seek to develop a therapeutic relationship with the group therapist, but not with the other group members. This may reflect a narcissistic need, or it may be related to other factors, such as not being accepted by the group. The tendency of a group member to speak to the therapist rather than to the group should be discouraged, as the power of group therapy is diminished when a person is simply receiving individual treatment with onlookers. In one instance, I had difficulty finding my way out of such a situation, and in fact it was not until too late that I had a more accurate perspective on the dynamics of the situation.

Manyara's group

Manyara was an African-American woman in her mid-30s who, after divorcing her abusive husband, had made a life for herself; she was working in a community nursing home and attending church. In a women's outpatient treatment program, she was effectively addressing her marijuana use, which she had perceived as becoming problematic. The other women in the art therapy group at the time were white and unemployed or dealing drugs; most had a longstanding methamphetamine use disorder; and most were involved in the criminal justice system. Manyara's striking looks and scrupulously micro-braided hairstyle were unintentionally alienating to her downtrodden-appearing cohort; in addition, her relative emotional stability and legitimate job status seemed to set her apart. Yet there seemed to be an unspoken feeling that being white was still the trump card in this group's cultural hierarchy.

Manyara's genial nature and occasional humorous remarks failed to cut the ice with her peers, who seemed stubbornly set to view her as some sort of cultural freak. For example, during a group discussion about setting boundaries with others, Manyara told the story of a predatory older man she had met at church, who "made his move" when her car wouldn't start after a service. At this point in her tale, Manyara quipped drily, "I looked up, and here come Sir Save-A-Ho on his white horse!" She grinned when I laughed spontaneously, but most of the group members literally just stared at her. Maintaining her equilibrium as usual, Manyara shrugged and proceeded to tell how she responded to the man's "bartering" proposal.

Toward the end of her last group session, Manyara doodled on a stray paper napkin as the group discussed the scheduled topic. Afterward, she handed me the serviette, with a throwaway line to the effect that since she hadn't got me a goodbye card, I could have this instead (see Figure 5.3). Looking at it later, my art therapy supervisor and I speculated that she felt lonely and ungrounded in sobriety and/or single life (water rather than solid ground under the house), and sought a way to connect to me (smoke toward the sun/observing eye) through the blockade of the rest of the group (firmly stitched-up white clouds). Her house/self looked confused or maybe even high/relapsing, with its X'd-out window eyes and tilt in the current as it drifted away.

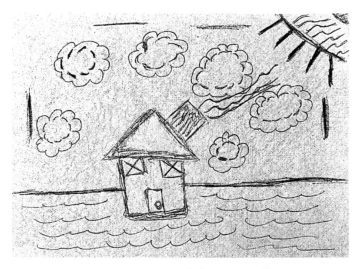

Figure 5.3: Manyara's "Goodbye card"

Perhaps, as so many clients do, Manyara had waited until she was out the door to share deeper personal feelings; and perhaps she was not even fully aware that she had done so. In hindsight, I felt I had not done enough to help the group explore and amend their behavior toward Manyara. The experience of universality and the building of tolerance and empathy toward others are benefits that might have accrued on both sides, had I done so.

Group member roles

Addressing the types of roles people assume in groups can help group members recognize these as a type of defense and as a personal stage that can be passed through. The shedding of personae or false identities enables group growth from the overly careful early stage to the later, more honest working stage. Groups can be taught about concepts such as the social microcosm, and how the dynamics of roles and transference create obstacles in communication.

In the time before the internet, fuzzy photocopies of an anonymous drawing made their way around self-help groups and treatment centers.

Captioned *The Group*, the drawing showed several men sitting in a circle, each characterized as a typical role in group therapy, such as the clown or the disengaged one. Since I was working in a women's treatment center at the time, I recreated the drawing, as shown in Figure 5.4, to depict women rather than men. I found that sharing this image was engaging and enlightening for clients; its humorous aspect was helpful in defusing discussion about these defensive roles. An associated activity is to have the clients draw their own in-group persona and accept feedback as to the accuracy of the self-depiction. Another option is to have group members find a collage image to represent their role in the group, and then to work together to place them all in a large collage. Using a structural systems approach, participants can experiment with placement and hypothesize how group relationships might influence individual change.

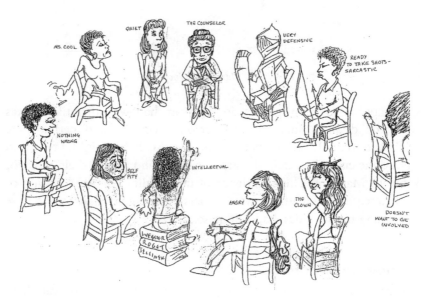

Figure 5.4: The women's group

Group art activities to enhance cohesion and ritual

Group activities that begin with individual art products that are then assembled to create a larger whole are relatively nonthreatening to make, and a satisfying metaphor for the group experience. Benefits are enhanced when the work can be displayed appropriately. In my experience, this type of activity has been instrumental in creating pride in the participants and providing inspiration for newcomers.

Paper wall quilts

One project involved building awareness of relapse triggers or barriers to recovery by first having group members brainstorm a master list (a sample list is given in Appendix A). Then, each person chose a personally meaningful trigger to illustrate colorfully on standard-size paper. These were then glued to a complementary color of larger construction paper, and the finished pieces assembled in a grid on black mural paper, allowing a black border to show between the pieces. The result was a striking-looking wall quilt that was gradually enlarged as participants thought of new additions. The quilt was used during group to discuss helpful responses to triggers. Next, a list of relapse prevention techniques was made and a corresponding quilt was pieced together as these solutions to triggers were generated. These ongoing projects provided a sense of continuity to treatment as new people rotated in and had unique ideas for the lists or unique ways to reconceptualize the drawings. The wall quilt concept can be used to illustrate a variety of other treatment concepts as well, such as things to be grateful for, or the Twelve Steps.

Graduation walls

Graduation rituals follow a longstanding tradition in SAT. The Valley Hope programs, which first opened in the late 1960s, have a tradition of encouraging each client to paint a ceramic coffee cup with a personal emblem of recovery. Painted cups are placed on special shelving at graduation, and graduates invited to return when they had achieved a year of sobriety, to retrieve their cup and share their story with those currently in treatment. An option that was popular with a residential women's treatment center also encouraged clients to return to share their story and pick up their image. In this case, it was an original or pre-drawn mandala coloring page that had negative space within the design to allow for words to be written. Participants would color the mandala, and in the space write an inspirational quote or words of encouragement for new clients. The client's date of graduation was noted in small print on the mandala before it was affixed to a black mural background with hook and loop tabs. When space needed to be made for a new graduate's mandala, the oldest mandala was removed and stored for that person's possible return. One person who had written the AA saying, "progress, not perfection" on her mandala discovered that, ironically, she had misspelled "perfection." She took this as a synchronicitous message, and rather than remaking the mandala, she drew a bandage over the error. These individualized portrayals of treatment wisdom create a more inspirational welcome for new clients than the same slogans on mass-produced posters.

Self-portrait flag line

This activity boosts morale by highlighting individuality as well as unity. Participants create a self-portrait using a starting prompt that is printed in very pale gray on cardstock (the template shown in Figure 5.5 has been darkened for visibility in this book). The use of a starting prompt provides reassurance to nonartists, and ensures that the finished product will appear more cohesive when attached. Two participants are given the templates for the two end figures, who are depicted as standard-bearers supporting each end of the flag line. Group size is flexible, as any number of people can receive the middle drawing. When the drawings are placed side by side, the figures appear to be holding hands or high-fiving.

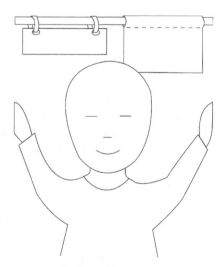

Figure 5.5: Flag line self-portrait drawing prompt

Participants are encouraged to choose drawing media they prefer, although they are reminded to consider the possible troublesome characteristics of their choice: marker pens are a difficult choice for skin tone and unyielding of mistakes; oil pastels can be messy; colored pencils may appear faded next to brighter media choices of neighboring participants. That said, participants are encouraged to focus on positive aspects, even humor, in their depiction, and not to worry about drawing ability. Clothing is decorated to portray individuality, and the two flags shown in each drawing are used to depict self symbols. Although some participants are initially unconfident about drawing their own faces, the faint prompt lines for placement of eyes, nose, and mouth are helpful. Most people enjoy identifying their favorite or fantasy clothes and symbols of things they like or that personify them. The completion of the task, either by posting along a wall or placing along the floor, often brings delight and good-natured laughter as participants see and share their images.

An option is for the residents to write their first name on the shirt or one of the flags. The flag line is pinned to the group wall, and incoming members are given the self-portrait activity as intake homework that they will add to the flag line in a group ritual. At a member's last group before completing treatment, a ritual is conducted of removing the self-portrait from the line and rebuilding the line so that it is unbroken. The graduating member can ask the group to sign the back of the image and take it home as a keepsake.

In a women's prison treatment setting, participants found it particularly satisfying to depict themselves in their favorite clothing styles, since they all had to wear the same uniform in prison. The group could readily be urged into discussion of what makes us individuals, which personal qualities are most important, and whether those can be viewed externally. In the prison, we could not post the pictures on the wall, but at the end of the session we laid them side by side on the floor along the wall, and took a gallery walk to experience our unified group.

This activity was also successful at an art therapy staff retreat provided for about a dozen administrators, counselors, and shift techs at a residential drug treatment center. For this use, participants were asked not to include their names on the images. Afterward, the flag line was posted along a hallway at the treatment center to demonstrate positive solidarity among staff. Additionally, a contest was created for the residents to guess the identity of the different staff; most didn't know many staff other than their own counselor. New residents were given numbered sheets corresponding to the numbered portraits and a scrambled list of staff names, and had to match the staff name to the correct self-portrait within their first four days. Since the staff were not particularly talented at depicting their own faces, they encouraged the new residents to informally interview them about their interests, in order to guess identities by the clothing or flag symbols.

This task gave residents a chance to feel more a part of the agency and to learn about each staff person, their role in the agency, and name. An unforeseen benefit was that it helped all staff get to know all the residents. The flag line game provided a humanistic, nonthreatening way for people to meet as individuals, whereas otherwise they might have pigeonholed each other as "the one with needle tracks" or "the kitchen worker." A sense of cohesion within the entire milieu is beneficial for worker morale, and treatment participants' positive identification with their agency, especially with a residential setting, supports a stronger recovery identity. Clients in such a setting are able to build a sense of having an alternate home and family—a sense of support that can be carried forward when they move back out into the world and begin to build new group and family relationships in recovery.

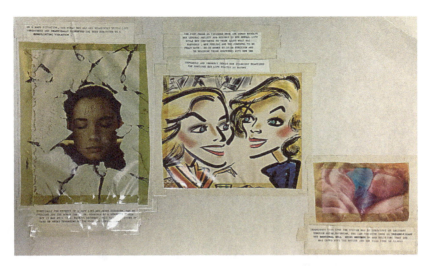

Figure P.1: Irene's collage. Irene used colored pencils to write words directly on the first image: on the woman's forehead, "DREAM," and on the shattered material surrounding her face, "ENORMOUS AGITATION," "SHOCK," "CRY + HYSTERIA," and "ANXIETY"

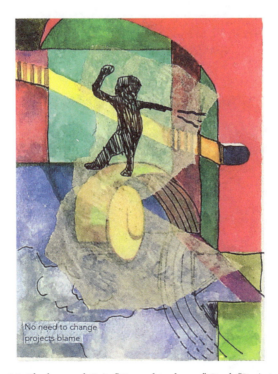

Figure 1.1: Shadow card. Suit: "No need to change." Card: "Projects blame"

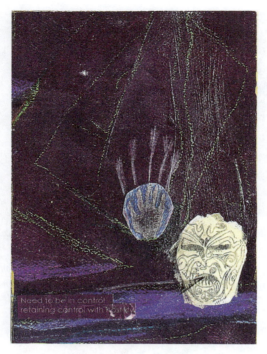

*Figure 1.2: Shadow card. Suit: "Need to be in control."
Card: "Retaining control with hostility"*

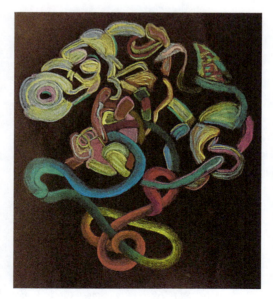

Figure 2.1: Alicia's "Brain on meth"

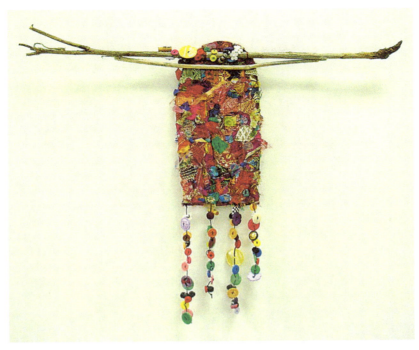

Figure 3.2: Rhoda's transformed wine bag

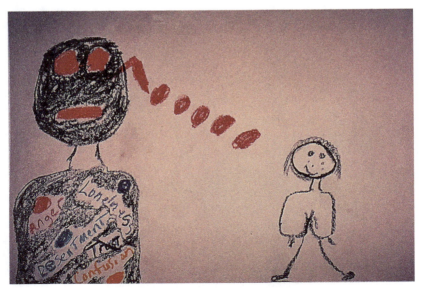

Figure 3.6: Martha and her son's feelings toward her

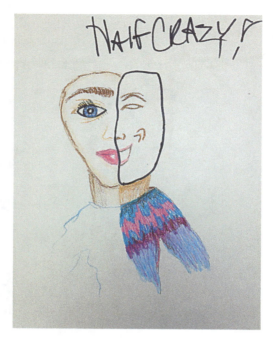

Figure 4.2: Marquette's half mask

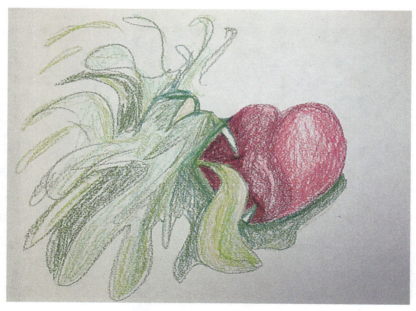

Figure 6.2: Teresa's second feelings-monster drawing: "Jealousy interacting with me"

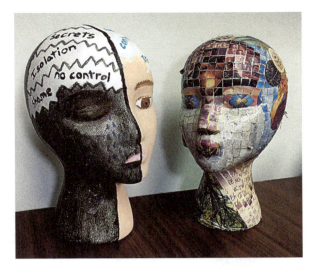

Figure 6.5: Heidi's (left) and the art therapist's (right) wig heads

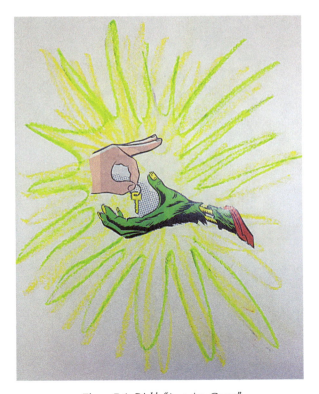

Figure 7.1: Rick's "Amazing Grace"

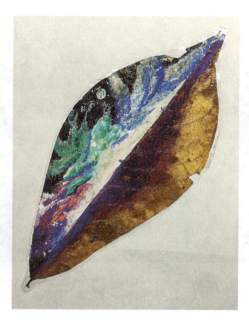

Figure 7.2: The cosmos in a pawpaw leaf

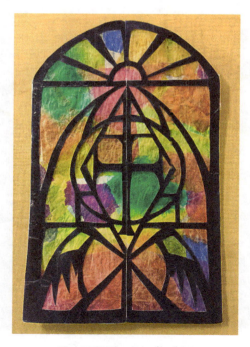

Figure 7.3: Secret garden doors

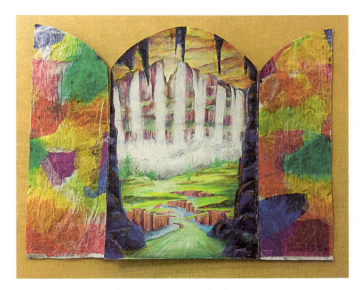

Figure 7.4: Secret garden interior

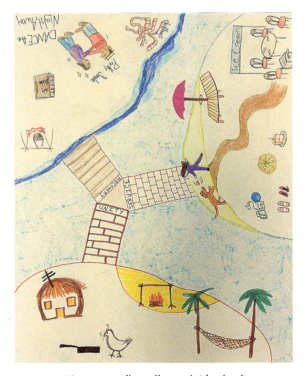

Figure 8.4: Al's small group's island task

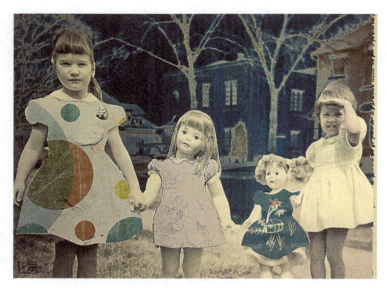

Figure 9.1: Photo collage: "Looking-good kids, guessing at what's normal"

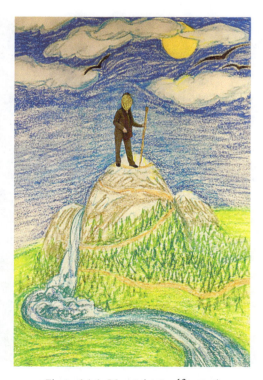

Figure AA.1: Mountaintop self-portrait

6

Feelings and Trauma

The incidence of untreated trauma is high among people with SUD, and suicide is a leading cause of death in this population (SAMHSA 2008). Substances are used to block painful feelings and memories; emotional problems and mood disorders may also result from addiction. The role of undesirable feelings in relapse must be addressed in treatment, and those in need of additional treatment for comorbid conditions must be identified and treated or referred appropriately. Although it is possible and often desirable to treat both addiction and conditions such as PTSD simultaneously, most SAT centers do not provide this kind of in-depth therapy.

People who have been suppressing their feelings may first need to learn to correctly identify them, and then, to appropriately respond to them. Early models of SAT sometimes forced clients to "feel their feelings" in group. Current trauma-informed practice emphasizes the creation of a safe setting and the establishment of trust in the therapeutic relationship or treatment group before processing emotions or traumatic material. Then, the emphasis is on learning emotional regulation by using mindfulness and relaxation techniques as well as learning skills in relationship communication and boundaries. Art therapy has the capacity to provide help all along the way, via catharsis, expressive communication, relaxation, and skill building.

This chapter provides directive ideas that correspond with common topics in feelings work, such as working through so-called negative feelings and learning to focus on positive ones. The intersection of substance abuse with childhood trauma, attachment, and sexual issues is explored, and a case vignette serves as an illustration of the application of art therapy to these concerns.

Approaches to feelings work

Feelings can be viewed as communications from the self about a person's condition, needs, and values in a given moment and situation. Most addicts have not allowed themselves to feel their feelings, whether out of pain and discomfort or fear that their resultant behavior would be out of control. In Martha's case (see Chapter 3), art therapy enabled *in vivo* exposure to feelings. Martha was encouraged to continue to draw her feelings after treatment to help maintain her ability to tolerate rather than repress them. Other contemplative methods such as meditation and mindfulness are used to "sit with" emotions. By regularly practicing interoceptive awareness—the consciousness of internal bodily states— clients can be more in tune with their personal emotional responses (Woodford 2012). This may be done by literally slowing down, breathing deeply, and trusting information from the gut or heart to guide our responses to emotional situations. This process in turn strengthens higher neural pathways related to emotional self-regulation and emotional development (Fosha, Siegel, and Solomon 2009).

Rational Emotive Behavior Therapy (REBT)

Variations of REBT (Ellis and Dryden 2007, first published 1997) are commonly taught in SAT programs. The foundational concept of this approach is that events or situations are not in themselves upsetting. Rather, it is our individual thoughts and feelings in response to those situations that color our perception of them, often resulting in undesirable behaviors and consequences.

The basis of the REBT approach is to identify reactive thoughts, then to challenge them by reframing the situation with different thoughts. It is helpful to provide concrete examples for clients, such as this: Driver A is driving on the highway and must come to a slow roll due to construction in the lanes ahead. He thinks about what a giant pain this is, starts fuming, and crowds the car in front of him. By the time he gets to his destination, the first thing he "needs" or "deserves" is a drink/drug. Meanwhile, Driver B, on the same stretch of road, sighs and thinks: Well, I guess this gives me a little extra time to think about my grocery list and listen to a book on tape; my plans might have to be adjusted or apologies made if I end up being late, but it is not the end of the world. The therapist points out that the situation itself is neutral; it is the drivers' thinking that creates an emotional experience.

Some clients are likely to protest that they are characterologically destined to react with rage when something stands in their way: "I want what I want when I want it" is an oft-heard phrase. The therapist can respond that human responses are more learned and habitual than inborn. This kind of work won't be equally easy or necessary for everyone, since some people have had good role models or are naturally more inclined to react calmly, but supporting belief in a permanently rageful or addictive personality destroys hope and stalls the change process. Assure clients that with practice, they can change their responses to everyday situations that previously led to acting out. New reactive thinking will become habitual if it is practiced, and they will begin to feel good about themselves for their new behaviors.

Reframing directive for REBT

The mental image of "reframing" thinking inspired the "no/halo" graphic art directive I developed for groups working on REBT skills. Participants use construction paper to make two circular frames: one black with a diagonal bar across it (the universal "no" mark), and one yellow, which is referred to as a halo. Setting these aside, each person thinks of a situation that has been predictably and problematically irritating or stressful for them. They devise a schema or symbol for it, and draw it twice, on separate sheets of paper. On one sheet, surrounding the symbol, the client writes all the thoughts and feelings that come up normally in response to that stimulus. Next, they think of counterstatements for each of the thoughts listed, and write them on the other drawing. The task ends by affirming the best options, by gluing or placing the "no" frame over the original responses and the "halo" frame over the reframed responses. The physical actions of writing out new thoughts, and the visual experience of affirming or denying the thoughts by framing them appropriately, reinforce and help internalize the learning.

Addressing negative feelings

A desire to escape feelings of anger, sadness, jealousy, fear, anxiety, shame, guilt, or grief may underlie the formation of an addiction habit, and clients often cite negative feelings as reasons for substance abuse. As part of the therapeutic conversation, therapists can ask whether, because a feeling is perceived as unpleasant, it should be labeled *negative*. Feelings can be reinterpreted as feedback provided by the body and mind about what needs to be experienced that will lead to healthy insight and change in the person's life. The ability to correctly identify, contain, and respond in a healthy way to the so-called negative feelings is also essential to avoid relapse. Therapeutic art tasks help clients explore and understand their feelings.

Anger: the iceberg and the volcano

The thought of their own anger can be threatening or curiosity-provoking for clients; some readily discuss it, whereas others completely deny experiencing it. "I never get angry" is a not-uncommon remark, but it is one that requires exploration. It may be true in that the person has anesthetized their anger and has never acted out in an angry way, but it is likely that once sober, angry feelings will surface. Being able to identify anger as a human experience, one that is rarely cause for panic or denial, is an important accomplishment. The therapist must be mindful that some clients may have experienced abuse at the hands of very angry people and have good reason to wish to deny the feeling, whether the anger is their own or another's. Some clients may be triggered by angry expressions by peers in group. It is important to be observant and help all members process their experience.

Anger often serves as a cover for deeper feelings, such as hurt, shame, rejection, abandonment, perceived injustice, sorrow, despair, or grief. For most people, anger is perceived as preferable to those feelings. The anger-iceberg directive idea has been handed around for many years and involves the concept of the anger being just the tip of the iceberg, while its primary mass, which is under the waterline and cannot be seen, contains the feelings beneath the anger. Asking clients to create their anger iceberg, or if preferred, an anger volcano, with the hidden feelings depicted inside the volcanic mountain or erupting uncontrollably, helps them picture and better understand this information. Sharing this type of art in a group increases the benefits, as clients will learn from each other. Participants might also explore whether their choice of an iceberg or a volcano reflected whether their feelings were feared, frozen, or volatile.

Jealousy: Teresa and the feelings-monster task

The feelings-monster task can be used with any problematic emotion. Teresa was a participant in a women's group that focused on relationship issues and shared troubling feelings of jealousy. She and her boyfriend liked to spend evenings at a favorite club, and she reported frequently becoming drunk to relieve painful jealousy from watching interactions between her boyfriend and other women. When she analyzed these behaviors objectively, she did not perceive them to be seriously flirtatious; her jealousy was more about her own feelings of inadequacy being triggered by women she believed to be more desirable. She stated that she would probably never really be comfortable when other women were in the same room with her and her boyfriend.

Participants were asked to create a three-part illustrated narrative about a personally threatening feeling, which is depicted as a monster. The intention of the feelings-monster directive is to help clients gain perspective on an internalized feeling by conceptualizing it as a separate being, and then to generate solutions from previously demonstrated strengths. With its narrative therapy and CBT properties, this directive has the advantage of being readily described in progress notes. Participants are asked to identify a challenging feeling and to make three images, depicting:

1. your troublesome feeling as a monster
2. the monster as it attacks or interacts with you, and
3. a time when you overcame the monster in some way.

Teresa was readily engaged in this task. She shared how her jealous feelings made her sick to her stomach, and described her jealousy monster as looking like green vomit with snake eyes and teeth (see Figure 6.1). She spoke of how she could feel jealousy squeezing her heart, and for her second picture, depicted the monster with its teeth firmly gripping a disembodied heart, a powerful self symbol for this task (see Figure 6.2). Initially Teresa related the heart to her love for her boyfriend, which was crippled by jealousy, but as she continued processing her series of drawings she came to another layer of understanding. In the final drawing, depicting a time when she overcame her jealousy, she created a valentine for herself, and the jealousy monster had shrunk until it lay helplessly in her open palm (see Figure 6.3). She recalled a time in a bar when her boyfriend was playing in a billiards tournament, which was avidly being watched by attractive female bar patrons. Teresa had had a sudden realization that the evening would make her crazy with jealousy, and that she would be sloppy drunk by the time the tournament had ended. She followed an impulse to excuse herself, and walked down the block to go to a movie she had been wanting to see. She emerged from the cinema with a feeling that her entire life had somehow been refreshed. Now, Teresa looked back at her second drawing and saw a different dynamic. The jealousy monster was able to grip her heart only when her love for herself was inadequate.

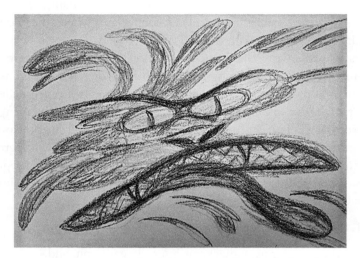

Figure 6.1: Teresa's first feelings-monster drawing: "Jealousy"

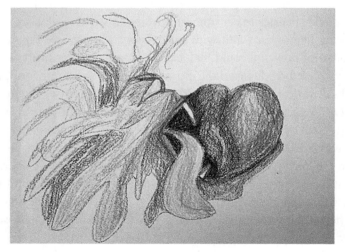

Figure 6.2: Teresa's second feelings-monster drawing: "Jealousy interacting with me" (see color plate)

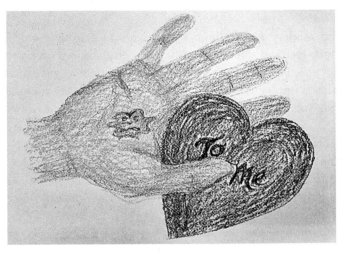

Figure 6.3: Teresa's third feelings-monster drawing: "A time I overcame Jealousy"

Fear and anxiety

Few people in SAT want to view their feelings of anxiety or dread as a form of fear, because being scared tends to be seen as a weakness of children. However, fear is often very real for people at this point in their lives, when the future is unknown and consequences of failure can be severe. Since clients will readily admit to being "stressed out," it can be helpful to reconceptualize this as experiencing the human emotion of fear during an important life transition. This can have the effect of elevating their experience to a grander level, which is somehow seen as more deserving of care. Groups who are asked to discuss fear will generally come to, or can be guided to, ways to handle fear, such as:

- naming the fear and having it heard by others
- getting more information about the thing that is feared
- hearing stories of others who got through a similar time of fear, and
- getting external reassurance and support.

They may recognize that these are the elements of learning and support that can be found in group art therapy and self-help groups such as AA.

Body maps

Fear and anxiety are feelings that often cause troublesome bodily symptoms. Helping clients identify their physical responses to these feelings can enable them to more readily use them as cues to become mindful and implement relapse prevention tactics. One time-honored technique for identifying bodily sensations and locations of feelings or ailments is body mapping (Liebmann 2004). Clients can be asked to use colors, lines, or symbols within the body outline to show where and how they feel fear. Then the same outline drawing could be used to show how the body feels when it is relaxed and soothed. A body-mapping task used to identify internal and external relapse triggers is provided in Appendix A.

Although some art therapists (e.g., Scott and Ross 2006) promote actual body tracing for this population, I do not recommend this, unless it is done by consensus in a group that has achieved a notable degree of maturity and cohesiveness (which might be possible in a long-stay residential setting, or in a closed-entry group in the later stages). Scott's recommendation to have clients choose the peer who traces them is a minimal safeguard. It can backfire when clients in early-stage treatment use this as an opportunity to flirt with someone, or conversely, are too fragile in new sobriety or with untreated sexual trauma to tolerate having this done by anyone at all. It is not enough for the facilitator to tell a group of people that they should speak up if they're not comfortable with the task; the individual who is truly feeling threatened is not likely to say so in the face of a therapist and peers who seem to be fine with the activity. A safer alternative is to use a generic body outline, which should be relatively realistic, as opposed to a cookie-cutter figure. These can be on regular paper, rather than life-sized; the art therapist could prepare in advance several alternatives of different human sizes and shapes, and also give clients the option of drawing their own.

Grief and loss

Grief issues are universal for people in SAT, although they may not be apparent at first. For some, grief is related to the addiction etiology: many began heavy drinking or other substance abuse due to a major loss or separation. Substance abuse disrupts the normal grieving process, and also enables denial of the need to grieve. When the person becomes sober, unresolved grief will likely return, although it may appear as anger, resentment, guilt, or depression—feelings also encountered during the normal grieving process.

Even clients whose original substance abuse was *not* provoked by loss are likely to create or encounter significant losses during the course of their addiction. These might be losses of relationships, monetary or property loss, health losses, job loss, and psychological losses (such as loss of time that could have been spent with children; loss of respect in the family, workplace, or community; or loss of self-esteem or self-confidence). However, rather than processing these losses as they come along, the substance abuse allows continued denial that anything is wrong, and blocks the sensation of sorrow, guilt, and other emotions related to grief. Even people who have suffered major or traumatic losses may be able to convince themselves and others that they have already grieved and coped successfully. Art therapists should be alert for signs of grief issues that may be projected in art products.

Ann's bridge drawing

Ann referred herself for treatment for alcohol dependence, and mentioned almost in passing to her intake counselor that she traced the initiation of her substance abuse to grieving the death of a child that had occurred a year previously when her husband had accidentally backed his pickup truck over their toddler in their driveway. His own grief and remorse had been intense, but soon he found himself managing the household and their older children virtually alone. Ann, unable to contain her grief or the rage that she knew was unfair to direct at her husband, had withdrawn into the bottle. She was now angry and resentful at having to give up this one source of solace, although she knew it was necessary.

Ann reached a turning point in her grieving process when she created a bridge drawing in group (see Figure 6.4). She had not yet shared the story of her loss with the other participants, although staff had encouraged her to do so. When she volunteered to share her bridge drawing, the tale came out; she looked at the drawing, held it up to show her peers, and spontaneously began talking about her child's death. She never referred to the drawing, but the sight of it as an illustration of her wretchedness amplified the emotion in her words.

The drawing seemed to compel the group to a compassionate rather than a judgmental response, which her story by itself would probably not have done. Ann was able to process a variety of negative feelings, including fear of committing suicide, also poignantly revealed in her drawing.

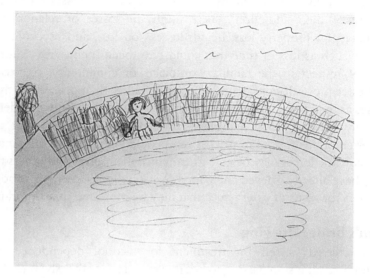

Figure 6.4: Ann's bridge drawing

Ann's story brings up a third factor that ties grief to SAT. This is the loss of the substance itself and its effect for the person. For most, their substance has been reliably on-call; whether it delivered oblivion, excitement, or capability, most people in early treatment believe that life will be forever horrible without it. Clients may also grieve the loss of the people, environment, or activities that may have to be relinquished along with the drug itself, due to their association and the likelihood that those elements would trigger relapse.

Grief counselors accept that each person has a personal timeline and way to grieve; this is no less true of people in SAT. It is important not to gloss over the process. Bellwood (1975) worked with grieving alcoholics in a special group wherein they engaged in "the constructive work of mourning" (p.8), which he enabled by fingerpainting and group exploration of emergent symbols or archetypes. Setting aside a special group and taking the time to go deeper can ensure more meaningful and lasting results.

Shame

It is essential to address issues of shame when working with people in SAT. Shame may not be evident in a client's initial presentation, but is often just under the surface. As denial begins to give way in treatment, painful feelings of guilt and regret may emerge. These feelings in turn cover a deeper nucleus of shame.

Shame is unique among the "feelings" in the strength of its tie to the core identity. It may be compounded by guilt-inducing personal actions or behaviors, but unlike guilt, shame concerns feelings of inferiority about who one is. Shame may also be compounded by clients' demographics or other characteristics beyond their control, such as poverty, physical unattractiveness, and traumatic experiences.

Guilt over past behaviors is usually an appropriate and useful response; shame is more deep-rooted and may have an existential quality. Many substance abusers feel that they are flawed at a very core level. Creativity and spirituality in therapy can bring healing to shame issues (L. Johnson, 1990; Wilson 2012). Shame issues can also be reframed using CBT approaches. The inner critic drawing (see Appendix A) is a directive that requires clients to personify and externalize their disparaging self-talk, which helps them gain the perspective needed to observe and challenge or disconnect from their own negativity.

Positive approaches

Hanson (2013) cited neurological evidence to encourage therapists to focus on helping clients devise "antidote experiences" (p.135) that strengthen the tendency to experience positive states. Chilton and Wilkinson (2015) described focusing on identifying positive emotions when working with people in substance abuse recovery. They asked clients to imagine their life in sobriety if it went as well as it possibly could. This imagining becomes a foundation for performing the traditional twelve step program advice to *fake it 'til you make it* and *act as if*. Positive emotions and actions not only reflect but also create wellbeing; they form a reinforcing loop. This is an important teaching point for this population, which tends to have a cynical view of positive thinking.

To prompt group discussion and individual art making in group, Chilton and Wilkinson (2015) used a list of ten positive emotions and associated ways of thinking, feeling, or behaving. The list was originally developed by Fredrickson (2009), who recommended mindful self-observation and striving for a ratio of three positive thoughts to each negative one. Items on the list include *interest* (noticing life's possibilities, feeling open and alive), *serenity* (mindful, peaceful savoring), *amusement, gratitude,* and *awe*. A blank board book or collage/mixed-media scrapbook makes a permanent container for personally meaningful images for each of these concepts. Other ideas from a positive art therapy approach include keeping a visual gratitude journal, or engaging in artwork depicting *you at your best* or *a pleasant visual memory* (Wilkinson and Chilton 2013, p.7).

Emotional regulation through activities

Flow is the name given by psychologist Csikszentmihalyi (1991) to the state of pleasant alertness attained during an activity wherein the brain is perceptive and calm. Productivity may seem effortless, and the person often loses track of time or awareness of surrounding distractions. This state is perceived as engaging to those who have abused drugs. Therapists can teach that stress-relieving benefits of flow are made possible by engaging in an active, rather than passive, reward activity, where success and mastery are enabled. When asked, many people will realize that much of their spare time is spent in passive reward activities, such as scrolling through their phone or watching TV.

Several variables contribute to the inducement of flow, but perhaps most important is that the challenge level of the task is properly aligned with the participant's skill level. The task should be neither too simple, which would lead to boredom, nor too difficult, which leads to frustration. Those who have a favorite hobby or craft are likely to identify its ability to put them in a flow state. One client with comorbid anxiety disorder carried colored gel pens and pieces of paper towel with her, and traced the embossed patterns on the towels with the colored pens to soothe herself. She described the excitement of finding a new brand or a seasonal design. After we had discussed flow in group, she theorized that the failure she sometimes experienced at being soothed could be due to the sameness of the pattern failing to provide enough challenge for her to achieve the flow state. She decided to start using intricate mandala coloring pages as well.

Teaching clients about the flow state can be easier than teaching meditation or mindfulness techniques, and its practice may have similar benefits. Gutman and Schindler (2007) discussed the neurological function of activities as a nonpharmaceutical way to regulate emotion and anxiety. In particular, repetitive motions appear to activate the parasympathetic nervous system, which quiets the stress response. One client of mine was able to tolerate processing angry feelings toward a parent by simultaneously performing the controlled stabbings of needle felting. Helping a client identify an activity that holds appeal is important; some may already recognize the value of an established hobby such as knitting, scrapbooking, or wood carving. Coloring pages, beading, or working with clay or papier-mâché can result in a flow experience for those who have no creative hobbies or are less skilled in art.

Trauma, attachment, and sexual issues

Clients' behavioral responses to traumatic experiences such as childhood abuse may involve delinquent or criminal behaviors as well as problematic substance use, both of which are under-identified as symptoms or consequences of trauma (Glidden and Brown, 2016). The historical response has been to punish rather than treat these behaviors, even when precipitating factors including trauma were known. Now that trauma-informed approaches to mental healthcare are considered best practice and legislative change is swinging toward the decriminalization of substance involvement, this situation is positively impacted. However, it remains a challenge to incorporate individualized trauma treatment into what is usually a highly structured SAT setting. Counselors' awareness of individual client needs is important; art therapists in particular need to be alert to signs of clients' trauma-related stress in art products, to devise appropriate responses, and communicate with other staff.

The impact of childhood trauma on adult post-traumatic stress disorder and substance use disorder

The correlation of childhood trauma to adult substance abuse has been demonstrated in several studies. Wu *et al.* (2010) found that greater exposure to childhood traumatic experiences significantly increased the odds of several adverse health outcomes in adulthood, including alcohol dependence and injection drug use. Similar findings have been reported by the ongoing Adverse Childhood Experiences (ACEs) study co-sponsored by the US Centers for Disease Control and Prevention (CDC), which identified childhood risk and resilience factors for adulthood diseases and conditions. Ten ACEs are identified as childhood experiences: physical, sexual, or emotional abuse; physical or emotional neglect; witnessing parental violence; having parents separate or divorce; and having a family member who abuses substances, has a mental illness, or is incarcerated. Among many findings, this study reported that a person who had four ACEs was five times more likely to be an alcoholic as an adult than someone who had none (Felitti *et al.* 1998; Glidden and Brown 2016).

Dore (2012) reported that 80 percent of clients being treated for substance abuse had experienced at least one category of trauma. Khoury *et al.* (2010) found strong links between childhood traumatization and SUDs, and their joint associations with adult PTSD. The authors suggested that providers should be aware of the comorbidity of PTSD and SUD in high-risk populations, and to consider appropriate treatment implications.

Attachment issues

Another contributing factor to addictive behavior is early attachment difficulty. Inattentive or unavailable caregiving results in anxious or avoidant attachment patterns in the infant, who then learns to perceive the world as untrustworthy or hostile (Bowlby 1988). Flores (2004) found that those with strong early attachment have less need of external sources of emotional regulation (such as drug-taking) as adults; conversely, substance abuse is a reparative attempt by those with poor early attachment that only serves to exacerbate characterological problems. Flores emphasized the importance of the therapeutic relationship in SAT, since it serves as a reparative attachment experience, but believed that group therapy was the treatment of choice for this population (Flores, 2004). Siporin (2010) observed that reparative attachment is implicit in the success of twelve step programs and of cohesively operating interpersonal group therapy.

Several art therapists, including Gerity (2001) and Kaiser and Deaver (2009), have referenced Winnicott's terms and concepts about the importance of the therapist recreating the role of a caregiver who creates a *holding environment* wherein the client can operate from a secure base with the mirroring approval of the parental object/therapist. Art therapy approaches and techniques are ideal for containing feelings and relating with clients in a supportive and admiring way, which enables reparative play and a sense of secure attachment. By filling in the gaps in early developmental experience, art therapists assist clients to function on a healthier adult level.

Loss of their drug of choice, which served neurologically and emotionally as an attachment substitute, will leave people in early recovery grasping for a replacement. When treatment providers and self-help fellowships fill the gap with secure relationships and rewarding processes such as art therapy, they help clients refrain from substitutes such as other drug or process addictions or unhealthy relationships. The phenomenon of treatment romance is a related issue for which therapists should prepare, and it is discussed in the next section.

Sexuality and substance abuse

Sexual issues are not always addressed directly in current treatment models, although this is a loaded issue for the population. Factors compounding these issues are often outside the person's control, such as early attachment deficits, ACEs, atypical gender identity or sexual orientation, and adverse adult sexual experiences. In addition, when they are actively under the influence, people may behave sexually in ways they would never consider doing otherwise. Upon becoming sober later, the person may feel alarmed and ashamed. The likelihood of being sexually victimized increases with substance abuse. Even before the new "date rape drugs" like Rohypnol® were known, getting someone drunk or high has been a time-honored means of expediting sexual victimization.

Another not-uncommon dynamic is that a person's values lapse as their addiction progresses, and they are more likely to readily engage in sexual behaviors that they would not have earlier, regardless of how drunk or high they are in the moment. This can include allowing themselves to be victimized, taking a perpetrator role, or simply being thoughtlessly promiscuous (Kasl 1989). Once in treatment, acts for which the person felt no shame at the time are often seen in another light.

The presence or level of victimization, culpability, and shame varies greatly in substance-use-related sexual encounters. Even in one individual, there may be multiple experiences of all these types. Cherished memories of high sex with a loved person may coexist with memories of shameful experiences. Some clients retreat into celibacy. Group work is a good way to normalize the variety of sexual issues and responses. However, particularly when working with groups, therapists should both be aware that some clients will not remember past experiences until they are sober, and watch for cues that memories are emerging or that deeper individual (or specialized group) work is needed. Clients need to be protected from over-exposing themselves in groups that are not intended to process past sexual trauma.

Processing past negative sexual experiences is only a beginning for most people in recovery. They will need to relearn sexual boundaries or learn to enjoy sex sober, without using a drug to reduce self-consciousness or to enhance libido. It is not unusual to hear clients say they have never had a sexual experience when they weren't high. This can create great anxiety about upcoming encounters after leaving treatment, even for those returning to long-term relationships (Mooney et al. 2014).

Another effect seen in clients in drug treatment is that when they have become abstinent, many have a renewed sexual drive. For others, sobriety brings a pink cloud of romantic feelings that may be readily projected onto a peer in treatment. Treatment romances, or cases of falling in love or lust that are particularly common in residential settings, are the bane of counselors trying to keep people focused. But like other seemingly problematic issues that arise in treatment, this can become grist for the mill, and in fact might provide an opening to broach the broader topic of sexuality in recovery.

Psychoeducational components can let clients know that having romantic or lustful feelings is normal in early sobriety, although that does not mean they should be acted upon. Findings of neuroscience have provided support for object relations explanations for addictive behavior. The actions of dopamine and oxytocin in brainstem and limbic functions are similar in positive attachment and intoxication; substance use may be a learned response to attachment deprivation because it satisfies the same brain function. Then, when the substance is no longer being used, a substitute is sought. This may be in the form of a love object (person) or of another activity, such as shopping, eating, or working (Bricker 2014).

By exploring these unromantic roots of treatment romance, clients having misguided early sobriety love affairs may be assisted back down to earth. Decisions about new relationships should wait until later in sobriety, when brain and behavior are back to normal. The wisdom of AA is that newcomers wait a year before becoming romantically involved. This might seem extreme, but most experienced therapists know of people in early recovery who were convinced they had found their soulmate, left their spouse and children, and later realized that they had made a foolish and irreversible mistake.

Treatment for substance abuse and trauma history

Research has supported the simultaneous treatment of substance abuse and co-occurring disorders including PTSD (NIDA 2012). However, the principles of trauma-informed care require that treatment planning be highly individualized. Just as with client-centered SAT planning, devising therapeutic goals and approaches for someone with trauma issues requires knowledge of the client's history and their input regarding what will help. Detoxification should be completed before the client is asked for a trauma history.

Sometimes a client will begin to share traumatic history before they are really ready. Art therapist and trauma expert Spring (1985) believed that clients needed to be sober for a minimum of six weeks before beginning to work on problems related to sexual abuse. She noted that some untreated trauma patients might not be able to maintain sobriety due to insufficient ego strength coupled with unrelenting emotional pain or flashbacks. Such a person needs to find acceptance and social support in a long-term caring environment with concurrent treatment of the trauma issues.

Skeffington and Browne (2014) described art therapy that enabled a woman to process a secret of familial incest that did not involve herself. This case occurred in a small women's-only art therapy group within a SAT program, which allowed participants to engage at their own level of comfort. The theme in this session was simply "childhood memories," and the client felt the support of the group as she began to describe her drawing of the childhood home and garden. Until she decided she felt safe making the disclosure, she could have characterized the drawing in whatever way she felt comfortable, although she herself was processing the reality at some level as she drew. As she processed her art, she made the revelation about the traumatic history. This example underscores the fact that there are a variety of experiences that people hold inside. Art making in a supportive environment allows people to gradually open the door to painful secrets that are otherwise likely to remain locked away.

Heidi revisited

Heidi's story has also been described in Chapter 2. The following vignette serves as a reminder that SAT groups need to be guided in a thoughtful manner. At one point while she was seeing me regularly for art therapy in my private practice, Heidi made the decision to attend an outpatient SAT program to address her reliance on alcohol. Our art therapy goals had been more focused on her trauma and anxiety issues, and she preferred not to have me serve as her addictions counselor as well.

In the co-ed outpatient program, she struggled with vague feelings that she didn't belong. She discussed her concerns appropriately with her individual counselor, and decided to persevere. A week or two later, the group counselor asked members to *share an unhappy childhood memory*. The culture at this agency was that complete participation was required of everyone. The intent of the request was probably to develop the ability to share deeper personal information and enhance the feeling of universality; most of the members were likely to have had adverse childhood experiences. But this request was in itself too provocative for someone who had been sexually, physically, and emotionally abused throughout her childhood. Heidi was flooded with an array of defensive feelings: shock, insult, rage. She left the group, and later explained to the staff that she had decided to discontinue treatment at the agency because she did not feel safe.

The addiction counselor who gave the group prompt may not have known about Heidi's trauma history, but this reinforces a point of creating safety for clients. I believe that therapists who work with this population must continually remind themselves that there are, more likely than not, clients in the room each day who have had intense experiences that have not been revealed or addressed. It is important for the therapist to imagine being in such a raw, newly sober condition. This will assist in devising ways to word directives in a nonthreatening manner, and to give alternatives to requiring full participation, acknowledging that not everyone will feel safe enough to process on demand. Negative consequences result when we command the revelation of secrets; the fundamental rule of trauma-informed care is to first create a sense of safety for the client, and then to identify and explore helpful processes together. In our art therapy sessions, Heidi was quite inventive about devising activities that would help her express herself and reveal her feelings.

One time, Heidi was inspired by an unpainted Styrofoam wig head that was on a shelf in my art therapy studio. When she asked to have it, she explained that she had been looking at the head's profile, which made her think of the two halves she perceived in herself when it came to her alcohol issues. Heidi often achieved elementary satisfaction on a kinesthetic-sensory level by using liquid craft acrylics to paint dimensional items like this. In this case, higher functioning was also involved as she analyzed elements of her addicted self, used color and symbols to convey meaning, and labeled the piece. Her choice of words described the elements of the dual aspects of her being: her safe, happy self and her anxious, addicted self.

Heidi often printed or painted words in her art products. When I first started working with her, being something of an image purist, I was tempted to discourage her from putting words on her art, but I came to realize the importance for her of *naming*. The concept that we need to identify a problem before it can be solved, or name a hurt before it can be healed, is acknowledged by a range of scientific and spiritual traditions. Heidi's trauma history was tied up in chaotic memories and responses, and putting labels on things was a helpful way to start building order and structure. It represented a developmental step up from the wordlessness of her abuse experience and the anguish she felt over her alcohol use. The positive side of her head included labels such as honesty, trust, family, it's okay, and 12 steps.

Heidi would become absorbed in her own work both during execution and afterward. She would sit quietly when done, gazing at her finished work and pondering its meaning. She often seemed to prefer to do this without comment by me. Sometimes she would take the object home to live with it for a while, or take it to show her talk therapist, before returning it to the studio. When Heidi returned her wig head, it spent several months in the studio turned face to face with one she liked that I had collaged much earlier, during supervision with Bob Ault (see Figure 6.5).

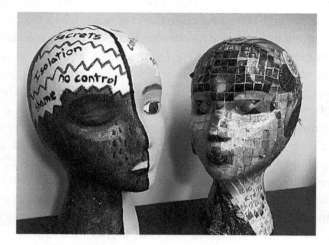

Figure 6.5: Heidi's (left) and the art therapist's (right) wig heads (see color plate)

These two heads, each with special meaning for us as individuals, together created a metaphorical tableau of my compassionate witnessing of Heidi's view of her diametric selves and her struggle to heal the split.

Heidi's story illustrates a point about finding the right treatment, particularly in cases where trauma is involved. For the client to feel safe is paramount, and identifying the best fit may require some experimentation. Heidi continued in her individual art therapy with me and talk therapy with her psychologist, and added a twelve step group, where she found an understanding sponsor, to work more actively on her drinking.

Conclusion: benefits of art therapy with feelings and relational issues

Art therapy has long been regarded as effective for working with trauma and feelings issues. These issues are often derived from or lead to problems with substance abuse. Art products and processing can be used to contain or express, to cathart or sublimate, in an overt or metaphorical manner, even without the client's conscious knowledge. In addition, art therapy activities can support and enhance the more cognitive behavioral and psychoeducational treatment approaches to relational and feelings issues that are promoted in SAT. The ability of art therapy to allow containment and metaphorical communication provides a safety feature for this work. In addition, triangulation with the art lessens defensiveness and transference, and allows for easier reparative attachment within the group or individual therapeutic relationship.

7
Spirituality

Many SAT programs offer segments or sessions that are allied with spiritual work, such as meditation or mindfulness, poetry, inspirational writing and myth, addiction-related cinema and music, dream work, and nature, in addition to emphasizing participation in AA or NA. Art therapists know that imagery makes abstract concepts more accessible; through art making, existential or spiritual concepts may be explored in a more satisfying way than with verbal attempts. This chapter examines the use of spiritual and related approaches in SAT along with specific topics that are frequently part of a curriculum. Vignettes and art exemplars highlight special techniques. The chapter concludes with a closer look at the philosophy of AA and the Twelve Steps.

Addiction, spirituality, and creativity

In a personal letter to AA co-founder Bill Wilson, Carl Jung wrote that an alcoholic's "spiritual thirst...for wholeness" is represented and subverted by craving and drinking alcohol. Having tried unsuccessfully to help an alcoholic through analysis, Jung condoned Wilson's approach, writing that "Alcohol in Latin is 'spiritus' and you use the same word for the highest religious experience as well as for the most depraving poison. The helpful formula therefore is: *spiritus contra spiritum*" (Jung 1963, p.1)—that is, spirituality counteracts alcoholism.

Writers including Leonard (1990), Grof (1993), and Cameron (2002) have also addressed the person whose unsatisfied spiritual longings are diverted through pursuit of chemically induced highs. These writers have suggested that one way out from this existential detour is to redirect the path of addiction by embodying the spiritual quest in creative pursuits. In a similar vein, Carolan (2007) referenced

Levine (1992) in suggesting that a relationship with the imaginal capacity is that which is desired, yet subverted, by people abusing substances. Without the capacity to create imagery, the person is hindered in understanding the unconscious on a personal or collective level. Art therapy can assist in transformation through the renovation of the imagination and the creative capacity. As described in Chapter 1, several other art therapists have published support of the application of creativity to spirituality and addiction issues.

Themes and techniques for encouraging spiritual exploration

The transformative effect of images

Lovell (2001) referred to imagery as a language that contains and expresses our physical and transpersonal realities, allowing us to experience that these two aspects are in essence indivisible. Most clients will acknowledge the existence of a part of themselves, and maybe also some universal presence, that are outside but tied to daily reality. However, they may hesitate to use the words *soul* or *God*. Concepts that are too religious sounding or difficult to express in words can instead be explored using stories and imagery. The therapist's own belief in the power of the image must be strong and conveyed to the clients. Inspirational posters are often found on the walls of treatment centers; quotations that reference imagery or creativity along with spirituality, such as Aristotle's "The soul doesn't think without an image," might be displayed on posters in the art therapy group room. These can serve as prompts for art responses in addition to increasing client awareness of more imaginal ways of conceptualizing spirituality.

Ecumenical author Rohr has written extensively about many spiritual topics, including the Twelve Steps (2011) and the role of imagery in spirituality. He has written that a flaw of the Protestant Reformation was its iconoclastic nature: the rejection of religious imagery and icons hinders the ability to access meaning on a deep level of knowing (Rohr 2015). Rohr referenced Jungian thought on archetypal imagery and transformation:

> Certain…images, art, and stories can have such a striking effect on you because what your unconscious has already half-known is brought home to conscious awareness by gazing upon them rather

than analyzing them. Analysis…is merely a control mechanism of the ego. *Let the images do something with you before you try to do something with them*… The great truths—when they can be visualized in images—reveal to you the deep patterns, and tell you that you are a part of the course of history and all humanity. That deeply heals you. It is less informational than transformational. (Rohr 2015, para.2, original emphasis)

Rick's "Amazing Grace"

Depict your higher power has been a popular art therapy directive in SAT. In an art therapy group session, Rick searched through a stack of old magazines and comics for an image he could relate to as a higher power. He had complained that he did not really believe in such a thing, at least, not in any way that he thought would be portrayed in a picture. However, he remained open to the attempt, and after a few minutes, he spotted and was intensely attracted to a large image in a comic book that showed a hand dropping a key into another, supplicating, zombie-like hand.

Rick carefully cut and glued the image to a piece of paper, and used leaf green and yellow crayons to create a radiating aura around it (see Figure 7.1). He then shared somewhat wonderingly about the experience this image had provoked. He told the group that he did not hold any particular religious beliefs but that when he first saw the image, he had the sensation that it represented the action of grace or being gifted with the key to recovery—that the only thing required on his part was the willingness to hold out his hand and accept the key. Personal merit was not required. The recipient's hand was not handsome or accessorized in a way that would symbolize worthiness—indeed, it was the hand of one who has suffered and is barely hanging on, that of the living dead. Rick went on to say that he had never particularly considered the words from "Amazing Grace" before, although he, like most people, had heard the 18th-century hymn many times ("Amazing grace…that saved a wretch like me"). He referred to the zombie hand as reminding him of the phrase *a wretch like me*. The metaphor was perfectly realized; to simply ask by reaching out one's hand, and to let go of control, to trust that the key will be given, is to be graced with the power to transform. For Rick, I believed it was not the words of the hymn that led to this deep knowing, but the imaginal capacity of his own soul, which was able to "think" in response to the synchronicitous appearance of this particular image.

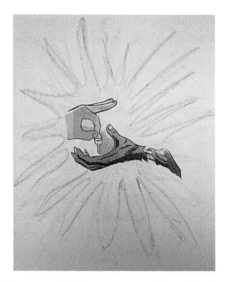

Figure 7.1: Rick's "Amazing Grace" (see color plate)

Inspirational readings

Despite the primary power of imagery, the power of words should not be discounted. Therapists working in a secular clinical setting may find it awkward to discuss spirituality, perhaps out of fear of crossing an ethical line into religious proselytizing, or of being discredited for being nonscientific. It is somewhat easier in SAT, due to the prevalence of the Twelve Steps philosophy. Often, clients are truly hungry to explore spiritual issues, but lack the words even to formulate the questions, or are too self-conscious to ask. Use of pocket-sized daily meditation books is a longstanding tradition in SAT. These are available on a variety of specific topics, such as recovery for adult children of alcoholics or for women with SUDs (see Appendix B). Excerpts from these and other inspirational writings can spur reflective art making as well as discussion. Participants can also be encouraged to share stories, books, or films that have personally inspired them in the past or that seem to hold new meaning for them as they embark on a new life path. Sometimes clients volunteer metaphors they have identified in popular literature or film. For example, Tolkien's *Lord of the Rings* hero Frodo's simultaneous loathing of and clutching to the burdensome ring of power is often cited by clients as a metaphor for addiction. The point is not whether they have accurately interpreted a writer or filmmaker's intention, but how metaphor in a certain work of art can hold powerful personal meaning and provide inspiration.

Dream work

Yalom (2009) recommended that therapists work with individual clients to "pillage and loot" dreams to access content that moves therapy forward (p.228). Moon (2007) developed a procedure for doing dream work in individual art therapy that uses a phenomenological approach to uncovering existential meaning. Doing dream work in SAT groups can be very meaningful, although it does not appeal to all clients and thus is most effective in optional sessions outside the curriculum. As with any particular approach, the therapist should be knowledgeable of doing this kind of work, particularly in groups, and have done personal work in this area. Therapists must not interpret for the client when it comes to dream work.

Nature and art therapy

The benefits of being outside in the natural world are apparent to anyone who has spent time with children there. Anxious energy diminishes and a sense of groundedness emerges. Adults in modern life may never take the opportunity to walk outside with no other purpose than to experience nature, but those who do often find it deeply healing and satisfying in what may be called a spiritual sense. Creating a visual journal based on natural observations is a way to honor this kind of experience. *Eco art therapy* seeks to engage participants with our primal bond with nature. Art therapist Speert (2016) cited the benefits of using natural found materials as art media, such as their varied sensory qualities, ability to build connection with seasonal cycles, and low or no cost. Eco art therapy frequently involves community, ritual, and interconnection, and thus has the potential to reduce depression, stigma, and isolation.

While walking in the woods with a friend, one artist was inspired to gather a fallen 12" pawpaw leaf. At home, she used it as a canvas for oil pastels to project an image of herself, represented by the green dot in the center of the leaf, standing in appreciation of the universe (see Figure 7.2). The finding of the leaf and the respectful use of it to convey appreciation of the natural world provided the artist with much-appreciated perspective on her life at the time, as she later reflected in her journal.

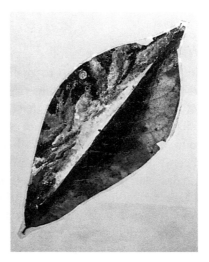

Figure 7.2: The cosmos in a pawpaw leaf (see color plate)

Mindfulness and similar approaches

Art therapists have applied mindfulness concepts to creative activities, and mindfulness practice is sometimes taught to clients in standard SAT. Prior to the arrival of mindfulness as currently defined, similar meditation techniques were taught. Mindfulness and biofeedback approaches are now being employed specifically to deal with triggers and cravings (Turner, Welches, and Conti 2013). A model called Mindfulness-based Relapse Prevention (MBRP) is showing promise in practice and research (Bowen, Chawla, and Marlatt 2011). In addition to these more practical benefits, mindfulness practices may raise spiritual awareness.

A defining practice of mindfulness is staying present in the moment—of being aware of one's thoughts, feelings, and actions as they are occurring. DuWors (2013) articulated how the teachings of AA employ many of the principles and techniques associated with mindfulness and other approaches such as Acceptance and Commitment Therapy (ACT), Dialectical Behavior Therapy (DBT), and Buddhist and yogic practices. Traditional treatment principles of taking life one day at a time and sitting with cravings until they pass are similar ideas to remaining present in the moment. The concept of surrender or letting go is another shared concept among these philosophies and practices.

Aesthetic art activities

Many SAT curriculums require participants to identify personal values. Art therapists can remind clients that the value of beauty, both of the natural world and of man-made items, is one that is often overlooked. Art appreciation activities can have therapeutic benefits when combined with group work, as has been described in the literature (e.g., Allen 1985; Feen-Calligan *et al.* 2008). Aesthetically well-done coloring page mandalas can provide sensory pleasure as well as a meditative process. Art tasks calling for depiction of safe places, places of beauty, or imagined other worlds can serve a similar function of providing both retreat and groundedness. Re-viewing or remembering the finished art product can serve as a mental safe haven at future stressful times.

When clients are creating their own art, art therapists can discuss helpful techniques:

- set an intention for their piece, in order to focus and then be receptive to whatever might come
- engage their senses with the media and allow for play or joy
- ask for technical help if needed to produce what is desired
- work with perceived mistakes and allow for serendipity, and
- leave their inner critics outside the door.

To create the secret garden directive as developed by Samantha Brandt (personal communication July 2015), participants fold the outer fourths of a large horizontally oriented paper inward, creating two doors. Inside, the client depicts a secret garden or other special place of serenity and peace. On the outside, the client illustrates the doors that guard it. One facilitator created an exemplar of this directive using colored tissue paper, a modified arch, and clear packaging tape to make the doors resemble stained glass windows that suggest religious symbolism (see Figure 7.3). However, when opened, they reveal a wonderful outdoor scene with waterfalls, stone, sky, and living foliage (see Figure 7.4). The meaning shifts, possibly to a spirituality that is reflected in the splendor of the natural world. The beautifully colored stained glass is a fitting but generic prelude to the richer, more personally meaningful domain.

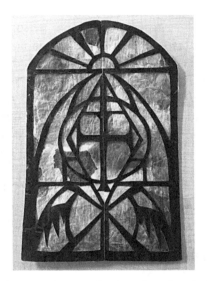

Figure 7.3: Secret garden doors (see color plate)

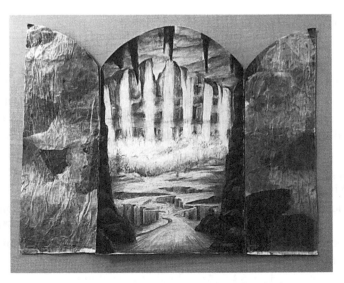

Figure 7.4: Secret garden interior (see color plate)

Special topics in addiction spirituality

Addiction is more than just an aspect of a person's life; it transforms the entire self. As one recovering person put it, addiction is like "a sentient being…living inside of you. Something you can't get rid of because killing it means killing you. But in dying you have a rebirth, a new life free from its control" (a recovering person, personal communication May 2015). I like this statement because it is not perfectly logical, and thus it more perfectly reflects the nature of addiction. People who experience the split, the being who lives inside, use every defense at their disposal to deny its existence and the need to let it die, which feels like a threat to the very self. As life consequences mount, the chronic user may attempt a partial intervention, or *half measure*, such as "I will only drink on weekends." But after a certain point in the progression of the addiction, some form of surrender must occur: either to the being that has subsumed the self, or to some alternate thing outside the self that might be called a higher power. Personal efforts having been ineffectual, the latter choice requires a leap of faith in that it involves letting go of control; however, it does not require that the person define a thing in which faith is invested. Especially as recovery begins, the higher power for many people is the drug treatment agency to which they relinquish themselves.

Acceptance of paradox

Whatever path of recovery is pursued, sooner or later an essential paradox arises: neither controlling nor letting go is sufficient to address addiction. Recovery requires an effort of will, yet willpower is not sufficient for recovery. It requires letting go, yet taking action, acknowledging powerlessness, yet performing with power. It might be said that both sides of the paradox are acknowledged in most treatment approaches today: spiritual or mindfulness practices, for letting go, and psychoeducational and cognitive behavioral techniques, for taking control.

Therapists working in SAT can expect clients who reject spiritual aspects of recovery because they fear, abhor, or simply cordially dislike "the God stuff." It is certainly possible to make use of nonspiritual means to recovery and be successful. Indeed, some still question the need for any kind of SAT. Anecdotal stories abound of people who just quit out of sheer doggedness, although they are often related by people invested in denial. Research has suggested that some people, particularly those who become addicted as a result of social behaviors in their early college years, simply "mature out" of their addictions (Stevens and Smith 2013). But most people in long-term recovery, whether or not they engaged in formal treatment or a twelve step program, will acknowledge the role of a deeper personal transformation that involved moral, existential, or spiritual change (Mooney *et al.* 2014).

Powerlessness and transformation

Understanding the neurological foundations of addiction, learning practical skills, and addressing feelings and trauma are all important elements of SAT. Yet the bottom line remains that to recover, a person must give up the compulsive attempts by the self or ego to control and manipulate a thing that is beyond its power to control. As the *Alcoholics Anonymous* authors put it, "Half measures availed us nothing"; "the result was nil until we let go absolutely" (AA 2001, first published 1939, pp.58–59). The path of change lies in relinquishing the illusion of control where control is impossible, but also of taking control— that is, taking positive action—in the arenas where action is possible. For the recovering person, it is not a question of total powerlessness or total power; it is knowing which is appropriate when. This concept is conveyed in a piece of writing commonly known as the "Serenity Prayer," probably written by theologian Reinhold Niebuhr, which is frequently referenced in SAT and twelve step programs in this form:

> *God grant me the serenity to accept the things I cannot change,*
> *the courage to change the things I can,*
> *and the wisdom to know the difference.*

Qualities of vulnerability, honesty, and humility are necessary for inner growth. Often these qualities are acquired from an experience of suffering or defeat. Rational thought and willpower are powerful processes of the mind, but crises of meaning and spiritual experiences may lead to the humility, letting go, and opening that are the means of deeper transformation.

Open-mindedness and humility

Closed-mindedness, which is often associated with the denial and narcissism of this population, stalls personal development. A popular, if crude, adage among recovering people is, "If you can't see how fucked up you are, you're going to keep getting fucked up." The path of recovery from addiction parallels the human journey from ignorance to self-realization. It begins, as it does for the fool on the journey of the tarot, with a naïve step off a cliff. Regaining the path rests on a realization that we, out of ignorance and not because of inherent evil, made choices that led to the highjacking of self that is addiction. Further, it helps to realize that we are not "God;" that is, we are not all-knowing and all-powerful. We didn't anticipate the cliff, and are unable to undo stepping off it. However, if we continue with an open mind instead of trying to scramble backwards to cling to our previous existence, we may find not only healing, but also treasures along the path ahead.

Progress, not perfection is a twelve step program slogan that encourages people to persevere in the forward movement, and to be humble and self-forgiving. The universality of the group experience ensures a realization that we are all human, have faults, and will never be perfect; that is how the world is, but we can forgive and it is okay. When working on these concepts in group, recall that metaphor, poetry, and stories make abstract concepts more accessible. Wisdom tales from many cultures and religious traditions tell of the beauty and spirituality of imperfection (Kurtz and Ketcham 1992). Such stories can serve as prompts for art response making in groups.

Gratitude

Gratitude may be defined as the acknowledgement that one possesses or expects to receive advantages. It involves feelings that can range from contentedness to bliss. Korb (2012) reviewed research and found support for the conventional wisdom that one cannot feel gratitude and stress simultaneously. Concepts about gratitude have been explored in positive psychology or the psychology of happiness; they have been a staple of self-help programs, as indicated in popular advice to have an *attitude of gratitude*. Gratitude need not be transitive; a person can feel grateful without being grateful *to* someone or something (such as God). In this sense, it is a good topic for groups that have members with a range of spiritual or religious preferences.

Gratitude as a group art therapy topic inspires ideas for activities. To start, clients can be asked to make a list of things for which they are grateful; it is helpful to supply a structure for the list, such as basic needs, friendships, health, strengths, life experiences, everyday moments, things that make you laugh, things gained from hardship, favorite foods, activities, etc. I have asked clients to start by brainstorming a list of 50 things that make them happy. Initially this seems impossible, but as they go along they are excited to see how the list expands. Once a list has provided some clarity, clients can write about one or more of the things on the list, create a collage of the feeling of gratitude, write a thank-you letter to someone who made an item possible, make a poster of things they are grateful for, draw or paint a picture that evokes gratitude, create a gratitude altered book or journal, and so forth.

Spiritual, not religious

Spiritual change is not dependent on any particular religious beliefs, although they may coexist. Most addiction treatment programs will make this point to clients. Many PWAI are disgusted with religion, for a range of reasons. Religious abuse is under-referenced in counselor training, but people with this childhood experience may be more likely to abuse substances as adults. In brief, this concept refers to children who are raised with strict observance to religious doctrine in families that are simultaneously violent, uncaring, or otherwise unhealthy; sometimes, the religion is used to support forms of child abuse. The result may be an adult who is either rigidly religious and anxiety-prone or rejecting of anything remotely religious in nature (Booth 1991).

In some personal religious constructs, God may be perceived as a benevolent Santa Claus-like figure, or as a harsh authoritarian parent, but in either case, as one who withholds, punishes, or rewards according to his judgment of one's moral virtue or behaviors. PWAI who have such a view of God may have difficulty feeling worthy of good things like a happy life in recovery. Another stuck point occurs when clients have rejected God, or decided he doesn't exist, because he failed to come to their aid when needed, or allowed a tragedy to befall: "He would have to be a real asshole to allow _____." Whatever the reason for aversion to religion, it is likely that these clients have prematurely rejected concepts that are more approachable in a spiritual context. In the process, they may be denying their own "thirst for wholeness."

Client resistance and other issues pertaining to Alcoholics Anonymous and Narcotics Anonymous

A well-considered understanding of these issues on the part of the therapist is important. Ethically, therapists must respect clients' religious identity or lack of it. But it is not necessary or helpful to capitulate at the first protest of "I don't want to go to AA, I don't believe in all that God stuff," when whether one believes in God is not an issue.

Not only are twelve step meetings and step work imbedded into many treatment programs, but referral to AA or NA in the community at discharge is also often considered the primary means for people to maintain abstinence and develop a recovery identity post-treatment. There is no cost to attend these twelve step groups, and they have helped millions of religiously diverse people to recover from addiction. Indeed, AA was devised as an alternative to a sobriety program that the AA founders judged to be too religious (Kurtz 2008). AA and NA encourage new members, atheists, and agnostics to remain open-minded and to *take what you need (or like) and leave the rest*. Material from the "Big Book" (*Alcoholics Anonymous*) that is read at the beginning of each meeting states that the only requirement for membership is a desire to stop drinking or using.

No one would deny that the Twelve Steps present spiritual and moral issues. Some of the frequently referenced slogans, rituals of individual groups, and steps do include religious language, such as the slogan "*Let Go—Let God*," or the tradition of some meetings to close by saying the Lord's Prayer (although this is nowhere officially recommended in the AA literature) (Mooney *et al.* 2014). However, twelve step programs do not promote the dogma or doctrine of any particular religious faith, and participants are not required to subscribe to any particular belief or to take part in any ritual they find disagreeable. A person who is working the steps is encouraged to come to believe in a higher power, thereby to let go of the belief that they can singlehandedly control the addiction. The freedom to *personally identify* a higher power, or what

AA historian and spiritual writer Kurtz called "some beyond" (White 2014, p.22), is at the very core of AA philosophy.

AA literature, and many treatment providers, suggest that a person can begin step work by using anything for their higher power, as long as it is not their own ego. "It could be a doorknob" is the phrase sometimes heard to get this idea across. A more meaningful choice might be the power of the AA fellowship. Treatment provider and writer LaPierre (2016) noted that resistance is almost always fear-based; he encourages PWAI to try AA by describing it as a group of helpful people with a shared problem:

> Going to an AA meeting allows one to consult informally with a room full of experts on what does and does not work for them individually and collectively. Plenty of folks in AA don't care for religion or rigid belief. They just found that they could not stay sober alone and they found that they needed to have faith in something more powerful than self. Some connect to nature, some to religion, some to spirituality, and some to a Group Of Drunks [G.O.D., slang for the AA group as higher power]. (para. 11)

The spirituality of AA involves storytelling. Members offer their own recovery tale to others, and in turn may absorb and incorporate what they hear of others into their own life in recovery (Kurtz, interviewed in White 2014). The sharing of stories is an integral part of the healing process. Hearing how others overcame their own resistance to change or acceptance of a higher power alleviates the anxiety of people in early recovery. Each person's story is different, and each person gains insight into their own journey by sharing with others who have faced similar challenges.

After exploring these issues, if a therapist believes that a client cannot make use of a spiritual approach, it is important not to also disregard the fellowship benefit of self-help groups, especially once the client is out of treatment and has lost the support of professional treatment. Although AA and NA remain the most geographically available recovery groups, several organizations have been developed as nonspiritual alternatives to AA and NA (see Appendix B for recommendations). Therapists can help clients find additional information online to determine the best fit, checking for groups that are geographically available or that provide online meetings.

The Twelve Steps

The Twelve Steps were first published in the "Big Book" of Alcoholics Anonymous in 1939. The founder of AA wrote that, "belief in them as they stand is not at all a requirement for membership among us…" (*Alcoholics Anonymous Comes of Age*, AA 2010, p.81, first published 1957). The original Twelve Steps have been adapted by Narcotics Anonymous, Cocaine Anonymous, and multiple other self-help groups. They have also been altered unofficially, such as by local groups reading the phrase "God as we understood Him" as "God as we understand God" to eliminate the gender pronoun. More than two dozen variations of the steps have been devised by various authors to address the specific needs of atheists, women, Native Americans, and various religions; there is even a humanist version created by B.F. Skinner. One source describes Step 4 as *courage* in the White Bison approach, *moral inventory* in the Judeo-Christian tradition, *the eightfold path* in Buddhism, and *righteousness* in Islam (C., 2012).

Many treatment centers require clients to complete worksheets or journals to address the first few of the Twelve Steps. While this is beneficial, it is also important to convey to clients that "working the steps" does not mean getting through a check-off list and considering it done. Rather, the steps represent a developmental process of understanding and change, and are frequently revisited as the person goes through recovery and gains further insight. The Twelve Steps serve as a template for personal growth that is satisfying and grounding work for many people in recovery; they can be taken well beyond an initial goal of achieving and maintaining sobriety.

The Twelve Steps are given here as published by Alcoholics Anonymous World Services (AAWS), followed by a brief commentary that I have written using the first person plural (as do the steps). Outside formal treatment, people seeking recovery go about step work in the best way for them, usually with the assistance of a *sponsor*, that is, another AA member who has acquired more experience in sobriety and agrees to mentor the newcomer. When used within drug treatment, step work may be more proscribed through use of worksheets. Art therapists can counterbalance the cookie-cutter approach by encouraging response art and devising appropriate themes, directives, and media options to explore specific steps.

The Twelve Steps of Alcoholics Anonymous

Step 1: We admitted we were powerless over alcohol—that our lives had become unmanageable.

Step 2: Came to believe that a Power greater than ourselves could restore us to sanity.

Step 3: Made a decision to turn our will and our lives over to the care of God *as we understood Him*.

Step 4: Made a searching and fearless moral inventory of ourselves.

Step 5: Admitted to God, to ourselves, and to another human being the exact nature of our wrongs.

Step 6: Were entirely ready to have God remove all these defects of character.

Step 7: Humbly asked Him to remove our shortcomings.

Step 8: Made a list of all persons we had harmed and became willing to make amends to them all.

Step 9: Made direct amends to such people wherever possible, except when to do so would injure them or others.

Step 10: Continued to take personal inventory, and when we were wrong, promptly admitted it.

Step 11: Sought through prayer and meditation to improve our conscious contact with God *as we understood Him*, praying only for knowledge of His will for us and the power to carry that out.

Step 12: Having had a spiritual awakening as the result of these steps, we tried to carry this message to alcoholics and to practice these principles in all our affairs.

(AA 2001, pp.59–60)

Step 1: Acknowledging that a problem has become unmanageable and affected our lives is the first step toward change. This step requires shedding of denial, minimization, and investment in being right, which are defenses against shame. Introducing ourselves as addicts or alcoholics in a twelve step meeting ends denial and engages the shame-reducing power of universality. It is a way of saying, "I'm through kidding myself; I'm here to work and heal, together with you all in this room."

Step 2: We must acknowledge that the repetition of unsuccessful attempts to control the uncontrollable addiction is "insane," that is, not based on reality or logic. By witnessing successfully recovering people in the meetings, we may be open to the possibility that *some beyond* could avail to bring us, too, to a saner and more fulfilling life. For each individual, the nature of that power can be learned over time; it does not usually arrive like a bolt from the blue. The step was intentionally and carefully worded "*Came* to believe…" to stress that this is a process of believing, understanding, and defining. It was not written, "We announced our belief that the Christian God would cure our addiction, and checked this step off our list."

Step 3: (Here and in Step 11, the founders used italics to emphasize individual definitions of a higher power.) This step requires that we decide to make a commitment to let go of control. It does not require that we do it overnight, nor does it specify the nature of that to which we are letting go, nor does it suggest that the turning over is a once-and-done process. The language reflects movement in the stages of change, from ambiguity about change, to a decision to change, through maintenance and perhaps even relapse. As has been observed of human nature and intentions to change, we must often start over again.

Step 4: This step is often worked as a written product to assess our behaviors, attitudes, and values, which have been influenced for the worse as the addiction has progressed. It is not meant to be a punitive exercise, but to assist in overcoming denial and preparing to change through further steps. One writer referred to Jungian terminology when he called this step "shadow boxing" (Rohr 2011, p.32). It is not about revealing one's "evil self," but about bringing to light the previously split and denied parts, or shadow, that have been deemed unacceptable. The more invested we have been in maintaining a false persona, the more difficult this step will be, but all the more necessary for that.

Step 5: The concept of confession is approved both within and outside religious constructs as a cleansing process that enables change. This step is often accomplished by sharing one's fourth step inventory with an AA acquaintance or religious clergy who, importantly, should act only as a witness, not as a therapist or a commentator. The person who "hears the fifth step" should also not be a friend or family member who has been a recipient of bad behavior or may not know the extent of it. People working this step have often been unaware of the degree to which suppression of these shadow parts and secrets has impacted their lives; the experience of working this step with honesty can be tremendously cathartic.

Step 6: The wording of this step reflects movement away from ambiguity about decision, yet it is also a step of relative inaction that incorporates the concept of letting go. It is much more difficult to achieve this kind of readiness than to pledge we will remove our defects ourselves. To illustrate the difference, people who apply for public funding for gambling treatment in some states are required to register with local casinos, agreeing that if they attempt to come on the premises, the police will be called to remove them. The difference between saying "I won't do that anymore," and giving a higher authority the power to remove the option makes this step very challenging.

Step 7: An important emphasis here is the concept of engaging with a higher power by revealing vulnerability in asking for help. The gain in humility and reduction of self-will is more important than pinpointing exactly which shortcomings might be removed or how. It may be said that by working these steps, our shortcomings are reduced; the relationship with a higher power can be the fuel for change.

Step 8: This is another step that stops short of complete action. The process of *becoming willing* may take time, and involves preparation for the next step. Letting go of minimization, blaming, and rationalization for personal past behaviors is required. People working this step also need to let go of resentment for harms done to them, or the desire for retribution.

Step 9: Amends may include personal apologies, letters (not text messages), the return of stolen goods or money, or other appropriate gestures. This step requires careful preparation, so that hints of blame or rationalization do not stain the apologies. It is also imperative to accurately judge whether an amend might injure someone. Modern concepts of transparency may lead people to think a victim's *right to know* trumps other considerations. But telling all is frequently more self-serving than otherwise. For example, telling a spouse about prior adultery that had been successfully hidden may relieve the teller's guilt, but little can be done to actually make amends for the past behavior, and the knowledge gained will henceforth be painful and demoralizing for the spouse. Working with a sponsor on a plan for this step is recommended.

Step 10: This step has often been contrasted with the fourth; while the fourth takes care of the past, the tenth provides ongoing self-assessment. It is closely related to the concept of mindfulness. Many people make a habit of taking daily inventory as a way of staying conscious of personal habits and behaviors. Allowing wrongs or half-efforts to pile up again can be an invitation to relapse.

Step 11: Although this step refers to prayer and meditation, these terms are undefined in the program in any particular religious sense. The point is to retain mindful awareness and communion with something beyond, rather than reverting to a state wherein denial can again take hold.

Step 12: A spiritual awakening is another term that is individually defined; it may involve a sudden revelation, a gradual growth of faith, a sense of being open to something like grace, or a newfound desire to be of service to those who still struggle. Existential awareness is deepened in doing this work, regardless of how a higher power is defined. A natural characteristic of successful recovery is that people are drawn to help others, and altruistic behavior results in profound healing for both giver and receiver.

Conclusion

Many people won't recognize the need for a spiritual life while still involved with their substance. People in early treatment may resist *the God stuff* or equate spirituality with religion. Since religion may be associated with formal and informal commandments that restrict behavior, ongoing and eternal judgment, the threat of everlasting punishment, and a God that is the ultimate in authority figures, it is understandable that a person with drug addiction would not be attracted to anything close to it! To soothe initial resistance, some recovering pundits repeat an old saying to newcomers, "Religion is for people who are afraid of hell; spirituality is for people who have already been through hell." The universality experienced in both twelve step fellowships and treatment groups can open the door to a different experience of spirituality, as the newcomer is surrounded by support of others who have also "been through hell" and will share how they made their way back.

Art therapists understand the limitations of words. Even with long-term participation in twelve step groups, the finding of meaning is never a clear-cut or linear process. An assumption is that meaning can be conceived and expressed within the verbal structure of language, but this requires that words stand in for abstract concepts that may be more readily felt or sensed than intellectually known. When art therapists fully trust in the nonverbal process of their work, they can enable clients to find spiritual meaning, and perhaps even to delight in that which remains a mystery.

8
Diversity and Special Populations

Training in cultural diversity and sensitivity is a requirement in the education and credentialing of most mental health professionals. Within the SAT field, dedicated treatment tracks and entire settings have been developed for people who use hypodermic needles (who have specific related concerns such as HIV/AIDS or the need for pain management), pregnant women, single women with children, people in correctional settings, people with comorbid diagnoses, including specialty tracks within that category, and those from the LGBTQ community. Treatment programming has also been tailored to meet the special needs of adolescent and geriatric age groups. It is beyond the scope of this book to address all of these issues and subpopulations, but this chapter does provide an introduction to adolescent treatment. The chapter begins with a brief overview of diversity approaches, including a directive to enable clients to more readily discuss these issues, and a case example of working cross-culturally.

Cultural considerations

The Art Therapy Credentials Board (ATCB) Code of Ethics, to which all ATCB-credentialed art therapists must adhere, states, "Art therapists will not discriminate against or refuse professional services to individuals or groups based on age, gender, gender identity, gender expression, sexual orientation, ethnicity, race, national origin, culture, marital/partnership status, language preference, socioeconomic status, citizenship or immigration status, disability, religion/spirituality, or any other basis" (ATCB 2016, p.3). The latest revision of the ethical code of NAADAC includes a dedicated section on principles of cultural diversity that requires addiction professionals to "demonstrate cultural humility" and "advocate for the needs of the diverse populations they serve" (NAADAC 2016, p.12). A chairperson of the NAADAC ethics committee expressed concern about political trends in the US that support the attitude that counselors do not have to treat those with identities, values, or behaviors different than their own, which results in reduced access to treatment for those most marginalized by society (Johnson 2016). It is an ethical imperative for those providing SAT, which may include art therapists, to refrain from imposing personal beliefs or values onto clients or their treatment.

When working with people of a different culture than their own, some therapists may rely on an ethnic-focused approach and end up overemphasizing the impact of clients' differences on their substance abuse issues, to the detriment of the treatment process. Others may insist on a universalist approach ("Differences don't matter, we're all the same inside"), which minimizes factors that are important. The best approach is to remain in open dialogue with each individual client, and to recognize that the importance assigned by a client to any cultural or other factor of identity or experience may differ from another's, and may also change with time. Some clients accept more personal responsibility for their addiction after gaining hope and a new perspective in treatment; others judge themselves too harshly, with resultant self-esteem problems, when in truth the impact of external factors was significant. A mature locus of control is achieved by recognizing the sometimes-unearned negative impact of external factors, while realizing that the way forward depends on accepting personal responsibility for change.

The ADDRESSING model directive

Hays' ADDRESSING model (2016, first published 1996) is a well-known multidimensional conceptualization of human differences. The word is an anagram that pinpoints various aspects of identity. I have incorporated the ADDRESSING list into a directive for individuals or groups that is useful as an assessment, as well as a way to explore societal and internalized stigma. My revision of the list adds the drug culture, where Hays' original model split the two types of disabilities between the two Ds. The list I use looks like this:

A—Age and generational influence

D—Developmental and acquired disabilities

D—Drug, drinking, or criminal subculture

R—Religion and spirituality

E—Ethnic and racial identity

S—Socioeconomic status

S—Sexual orientation

I—Indigenous heritage

N—National origin

G—Gender and gender identity

(adapted from Hays 2016)

Clients are given a copy of the list and asked to think about how these factors have affected their life and substance use. They then identify the item that is most impactful for them at the current time, and use art materials to depict their feelings about it. The act of drawing or collaging about this characteristic can reveal deep-seated shame or anger. Discussion can explore power differentials in our society and how each of the ADDRESSING characteristics has the potential to empower or disempower an individual. Clients are usually quick to identify these dynamics. The therapist can ask, "How does the knowledge of personal powerlessness over this item, or the shame from an internalized sense of powerlessness, affect your substance use? Is it possible for the factor, or your perception of its importance, to be changed or modified in a positive way?" These discussions assist clients in accurately perceiving how factors of identity may be involved in their substance use, and establish which of these may need to be addressed for successful recovery.

The Replication, Re-vision, and Reflection (RRR) technique

Imagery can also help us see beyond cultural or other aspects of identity. A time-honored way for art therapists to process information outside the treatment session is to redraw client artwork or make response art. I developed the RRR as a way to achieve perspective and move past countertransference, which may be sparked by differences. The procedure is to be performed by the therapist alone. It involves copying a client's drawing as accurately as possible while observing internal responses; making a new, revised drawing that creates a more positive condition or outlook or resolves questionable content; and reflecting on the process in writing or verbally with a supervisor. Results must be interpreted with caution, as it is possible that projection and countertransference will continue to be enabled. Full directions are given in Appendix A.

The RRR has the potential to shed light on countertransference and reveal the client behind the treatment persona, whether the latter involves bravado, denial, clowning, or flight into health. It can help identify level of motivation, personal strengths, and direction for treatment planning.

An example of working cross-culturally: the case of Al

One of the most memorable times I used the RRR was when I worked in a residential substance abuse program as an art therapist who was also licensed as a substance abuse counselor. "Al" was an African-American man who identified as being of the "street" drug culture. Exploring Al's drawing led me to sense the alienation he might have felt in this program, which was staffed by white females and was middle class in its culture. Use of the RRR also helped me to see beyond Al's genial treatment persona.

Al was a small, wiry man in his mid-40s who stated he had reached the point in life where he was "sick and tired of being sick and tired" from his drug usage. He seemed earnestly to want to quit; he was in treatment without any legal contingencies. Al's primary defensive behavior was his charming and self-possessed, yet self-deprecating, sense of humor. Although treatment staff speculated that Al would retreat into humor as a defense against participating on a deeper level, it was difficult for anyone to challenge him on this point, because staff and residents alike enjoyed his happy and funny persona.

Looking back after doing the RRR, I realized I was guilty of supporting his mascot role and forgetting to look past Al's charm.

I scarcely noticed the potentially disturbing elements in his bridge drawing when he drew it in a group session, because I was distracted by his humorous play-by-play comments on his drawing ability. He expertly limited his comments to keep the group ambiance pleasant, without being disruptive. Further, when he shared his brief, unimaginative bridge story, I thought of it as the product of a concrete cognitive style; at the time, I did not consider that its generic terseness served to keep the lid on any deeper issues.

The RRR process with Al's bridge drawing

As I performed the RRR, the process of redrawing Al's figure on the bridge literally seemed to hit me in my core (see Figures 8.1 and 8.2). I felt vulnerable and incapable; it was a pathetic, lost-child feeling. When I had completed the figure, I found myself going back and retracing its outlines, as he had done, as if that would strengthen its boundaries and shield it. Then, when I drew the upper vertical supports for the bridge, I felt confusion and frustration. If I had verbalized the feeling, it might have been to say, "I know these things are supposed to uphold this bridge, but I can't get them to make sense!" That was when I truly realized how unlikely it was that Al, a black heroin user from the streets, would feel as understood by this program as would the white, white-collar men and women with alcohol problems who made up the majority of his cohort. The treatment structure he was in, his bridge, was not fully supporting his reality.

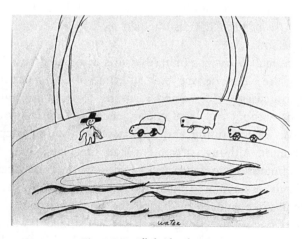

Figure 8.1: Al's bridge drawing

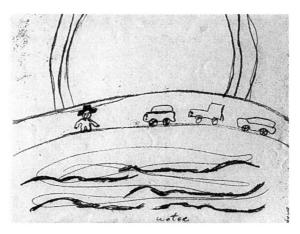

Figure 8.2: My replication of Al's bridge drawing

Remembering that Al had drawn the water last, with the darker wave lines on top, I did so too in my recreation. During group I had thought them odd, but Al had been chuckling softly as his tablemates watched, "Oh yeah, ya'll, these are waves...see, I can't even draw water!" At that point, in a humorous belabored manner, he had labeled the area with the word "water" (which is also slang for various illicit drugs, perhaps another joke). When I duplicated his lines, I found that it was relaxing. The heavier wavy lines felt good to make and I thought perhaps for that reason he had perseverated on them, especially if he had at first experienced feelings of ineffectualness and confusion, as I had earlier in the drawing. Perhaps the relaxed feeling echoed the way Al self-soothed with his drug of choice. In all his drawing/world, the water/drug may have been his only solace, the only thing he felt capable of manipulating in his environment that would make him feel good. Of course, comforting or compelling water beneath a bridge may also invoke thoughts of suicide to those so inclined, an option supported by the stance of the disempowered figure at the brink.

As I prepared to create a re-vision drawing, I literally felt a surge of relief at the return of my own sense of capability and control. This was accompanied by a more analytical, rather than emotional, brain functioning. I readily left behind the unpleasant feelings, made a mental list of drawing elements I wanted to correct, and planned the way I would lay out the drawing changes. This abrupt shift to left-brain functioning was amusing to reflect upon later, but it was also informative, for it seemed to suggest that power lay in a treatment focus *away* from the usual mandate to "feel your feelings." Perhaps rather than forcing Al to access those feelings he was avoiding, which might have involved despair and depression, we needed to help him experience a greater sense of capability. Empowerment might be gained by identifying new thoughts and behaviors and by cognitively mapping the structure of a new life in sobriety. Essential underlying support for this could be achieved through more transparent therapeutic relationships with staff and more caring interactions with all peers in the various groups, regardless of life experience.

In the Re-vision, I placed Al's figure on a sidewalk with a railing, dressed it, had it walking across the bridge rather than standing at the precipice, and turning to give the viewer a jaunty, self-confident wave (see Figure 8.3). As I drew, I thought, this is a way I could actually envision Al, at least in one alternative future. I found that I wasn't exactly sure how to design the bridge (his treatment plan) either, but attempted to make a more sensible and secure structure. I made Al move with the flow of traffic—toward the future, merging with the world at large to the extent necessary, rather than about to be run over, as in his drawing. I removed his fancy wheel covers (a detail he had pointed out in his drawing, which I chose to treat as a symbol of artificial values) to reveal serviceable black wall tires. I tried to depict the river flowing by, rather than waiting ominously, with its comforting but all-enveloping waves, for him to jump into oblivion. Finally, I added a whimsical fish poking out of the water as a symbol of his humor, which I regarded as a legitimate personal strength.

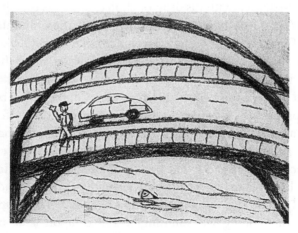

Figure 8.3: My Re-vision of Al's bridge drawing

A refreshed treatment approach

After performing the RRR, I shared my insights with the rest of the clinical team. We agreed that regardless of the accuracy of my feelings when redrawing Al's bridge world, my thoughts regarding possible interventions were legitimate enough to inform our approach with him. We did not change his treatment plan *per se*, but worked with him more transparently about challenges he might be facing in terms of case management. We also sought to stimulate group cohesion however possible, which would benefit not only Al but also all the clients. We hoped that if Al was able to experience a rewarding sense of fellowship with this cohort of addicts, most of whom were not otherwise much like him, he would be more likely to sample a variety of self-help groups in the community after discharge.

Al's last session: the group islands task

I had the previously stated goal in mind when I asked the participants in Al's last art therapy group session to do a group islands directive, which requires groups to work together on a single piece of poster board (22" × 28"). This represents the sea, and each participant creates their own island that contains their bare essentials for a happy life. The group met in the cafeteria and worked at 48" round tables; participants worked in subgroups of two to four at each table. Al's tablemates included Darlene, an outgoing African-American woman in her late 30s who had successfully completed treatment previously and was self-referred after having relapsed, and Brooke, a quiet Caucasian 19-year-old who was just starting treatment and seemed eager to please the counselors and do everything correctly. As was typical, the groups were silent when beginning their art work, but gradually and sporadically began to chat among themselves. (Although with some groups or directives it may be preferable not to allow talking during art making, it was allowed in our group culture, as long as talk did not turn to gossip, war stories, or was too loud or otherwise distracting.) Al's habitual complaints about being required to draw had become an ongoing group joke that he enjoyed perpetuating. When the island drawing directive was described, he laughed ironically, "Oh, here we go!" In actuality, I had noticed that he had been drawing more avidly and imaginatively with each opportunity.

Al's island (see Figure 8.4) depicts a snug thatched cottage with an old-fashioned TV antenna, a hammock between palm trees, a fire with a cooking spit on the beach, and a large frying pan with a chicken that seems to be peering into it uncomprehendingly. Al joked that he was good at making fried chicken, but that did not mean he could *draw* a chicken. He said that when he saw how well Brooke had drawn her pizza and shoes, he had asked for her help. He attracted my attention to this report with a grin and a fist pump, since it was on his treatment plan to practice becoming more comfortable asking others for help. Brooke had been happy to assist; she had drawn a chicken on a napkin, which he had then copied onto his island. Meantime, Darlene, who enjoyed drawing, featured herself "dancing the night away" with her husband, who is depicted with the label "pretty smile." Her island also included two other things she stated she couldn't live without: a Bible, labeled "JESUS" on the spine, and in the corner of the island, chitterlings awaiting the pot. She had carefully labeled the food while making a humorous remark about it, in a way that echoed and teased Al for ostentatiously labeling the water in his bridge drawing of a previous group.

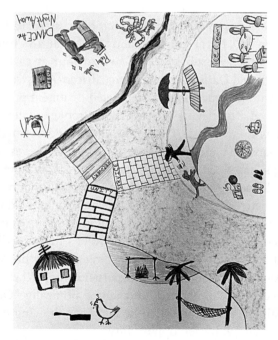

Figure 8.4: Al's small group's island task (see color plate)

Brooke seemed quite comfortable with the two older African-Americans at her table. Darlene seemed to take a motherly aspect toward her, and they shared a box of colored pencils and commented on each other's drawings as they drew. After observing Darlene's depiction of herself dancing with her husband, Brooke carefully depicted herself and her dog playing frisbee on the beach. At the facilitator's suggestion that people might want to visit each other's islands, Brooke ventured to Al and Darlene, "I could make an ice cream store for you guys to visit when you're done cooking!" It seemed to me a perfect childlike remark, with its unconscious compliment or appeal to Al and Darlene for their parental nurturing potential.

Darlene shaded the water with pastel and laid out the boardwalk to connect their islands. My attention was divided with multiple tables, but someone in this group noticed the triangle that resulted where their boardwalks met, and was inspired to add the three words that surround the triangle found in the AA logo: unity, service, recovery. As the session came to a close, Darlene spontaneously began to sing "Lean On Me" in a clear alto. Her tablemates and a few others in the room joined in: it was a classic community rehab moment, and I could not have wished for a better closure for Al's last session. The group islands activity embodied a message to Al that his own world could stay his own, yet coexist with others' in a satisfying, mutually supportive relationship.

Adolescents

While some therapists are drawn to work with this age group, many abhor it, or think they would. It is normal for adults to squirm when asked to recall those days or when debating whether to attend a class reunion; the teen years provide rich fodder for countertransference in that they were usually packed with emotion and not remembered with accurate perspective. In my personal experience, being the parent of an adolescent was the best training; it allowed me to reframe my personal history, normalize the population, and experience empathy much more deeply than I had previously. Those who lack adult life experience with this age group will be able to learn by doing, if they keep an open mind and seek reality checks from supervisors.

Normal developmental issues

Knowledge of adolescent development is essential. Typically developing adolescents possess the following characteristics, to varying degrees:

- self-centeredness, sense of entitlement
- struggles with authority figures, whether internal or overt
- judgmental toward status quo, world of adults
- activation of the personal fable ("I am unique, consequences won't apply")
- risk-taking behavior, unmindful of consequences
- avoidance of responsibility or guilt ("everyone does it")
- hyper-critical of select peers, self, younger children ("so stupid")
- over-identification with admired peers or celebrities (must mimic clothing, etc.)
- mood swings: hormonal changes and a still-developing brain result in the appearance of emotion ruling over intellect (limbic over cortical processing)
- speed of concrete cognitive processing dominates over slower, more analytical thinking that perceives patterns and consequences.

(adapted from Schmanke 2015)

If work with adolescents is not developmentally informed, therapists are sure to pathologize even normal behaviors. When mental, emotional, and behavioral patterns *are* atypical or diagnosable, continuing to view them through a developmental lens will ensure accurate expectations, facilitate the therapeutic relationship, inform treatment planning, and increase hope for recovery. Personal identity evolves throughout life, but the active search for identity often peaks during adolescence. Erikson's (1994, first published 1959) developmental predicaments of *identity vs. role confusion* and *intimacy vs. isolation* are active throughout the mid- and late teens and 20s, and are vastly complicated and prolonged by substance abuse. For girls or women and those in some nondominant cultures, relational issues may dominate or share the spotlight with the identity search.

Developmental tasks are bound up in a dynamic with the normal narcissism of adolescence and by the surge in creativity found in this age group. Blos (1962) described the adolescent creative drive as springing from the need to do the work of internal identity transformation, and remarked that adolescent artistic productions are often undisguisedly autobiographical. He observed that the creative process enhances adolescent "infatuation with the self" and the "conviction of being a chosen and special person" (Blos 1962, p.126), that is, the personal fable. Adolescents from impoverished or adverse environments or with substance use problems may carry a damaged personal fable, seeing themselves as hopeless or good for nothing; some may revel in this identity. Positively impacting the personal fable via art making that is syntonic with adolescent creativity can correct low self-esteem and inappropriate external locus of control.

Carolan (2007) postulated that the dominant culture's pressure for a linear process of development toward a rational, socially preferred identity results in repression of imaginal processes. Thus, adolescents who use substances may be unconsciously addressing the needs of the imaginal self. The role of art therapy in supplanting this need is obvious. Art tasks or themes that involve self-portraits or self-description are effective at holding interest and building identity.

Adolescent substance abuse issues
Etiology

Etiological factors for substance abuse that are unique to adolescence include the risk taking enabled by the personal fable (Alberts, Elkind, and Ginsberg 2007); peer pressure to use AOD; and easy availability despite legal constraints for minors (Tait 2013). As discussed in Chapter 6, the experience of childhood trauma (ACEs) is seen as a precursor to substance abuse. Adolescents are especially vulnerable to ongoing trauma and abuse in the home, due to their limited resources to live independently. And whether they are living on the street or in an elite boarding school, many adolescent PWAI lack an emotionally stable and supportive home.

Many adolescents turn to substance use to mask feelings of despair, fear, anger, and grief. In addition, many engage in self-harm and reckless behaviors of all kinds. The combination of behaviors may be pathologized and the substance-using adolescent dually diagnosed with bipolar disorder, ADHD, borderline personality, conduct disorder, or other diagnoses; this is not always helpful. When illicit drug use and reckless behaviors are not under control, there is a risk that prescribing psychiatric medication will only complicate matters. Teen clients are not likely to be compliant with their medications; indeed, many sell or trade their prescription medications for their drug of choice.

Resistance

Because conflict with authority is a developmental, not pathological, issue, therapists can count on adolescent clients to display resistance of varying kinds. When they are asked about their AOD use, most adolescents will minimize it, or use that favorite defense of early adolescence, "everyone does it" (which becomes convincing after one has been working in the field, but is far from true!). Some will exaggerate the extent of their use in a kind of bravado, or defiantly proclaim their intention to keep using and die young. Some are resistant by being physically aggressive; others refuse to participate. Many adolescents are simply shy; they have used drugs to feel comfortable in social situations, and missed out on developmental experiences to practice social communication while sober.

Drama therapist Emunah once wrote a phrase about working with adolescents that has supported me over the years: "Just beyond the resistance lies a readiness" (1990, p.101). If the therapist is patient, or at least does not reveal impatience, a trusting relationship is built and is there when the client is ready. The use of arts activities to triangulate the stress of the relationship allows adolescents to pass through an initial artistic response of explosion (catharsis), to more formed expression and containment, and finally to expansion (sublimation and communication) (Emunah 1990).

Resilience

Protective factors against substance abuse can ensure that adolescents do not go on to become addicted adults. In addition to identifying protective factors in the environment, such as a supportive family, school, and community, research has shown that adolescents with strong *resilience skills* are less likely to turn to AOD use either initially or after treatment (Tait 2013). Increased resilience involves learning or enhancing qualities such as hope and optimism, emotional and behavioral self-regulation, problem-solving skills, and a sense of humor.

Art therapists who design processes around these factors will boost their adolescent clients' chances for sustained recovery.

Use of combined theoretical approaches in art therapy treatment

The art therapist working with adolescents in SAT will want to consider approaches helpful for adolescents and incorporate these concepts into the agency substance abuse model. Riley (1999b) proposed a triangular model of treatment for adolescents, with the base being art therapy and the two sides representing adolescent developmental theory and a brief therapy model. She pointed out that adolescents are never eager for prolonged therapy, and respond best to a brief model that builds on strengths and identifies goals and interventions that are meaningful to the client.

Making the therapy meaningful to the client is particularly important when working with adolescents in treatment for SUD. Upon arrival, the client is unlikely to think that their substance use is problematic. The therapist must acknowledge the purpose of treatment, but also work with the client to identify problem areas and incorporate goals that they would find attractive. Often the very act of identifying these issues results in a new perspective about how much and in what ways the adolescent is capable of controlling their life, as well as the extent of the impact of their substance use on other life areas. A Motivational Interviewing (MI) approach will be most effective.

Riley (1999a, 1999b) borrowed concepts from a narrative approach as well. The developmental characteristic of being self-centered is readily addressed with art tasks reflecting the personal story. Her idea of making contrasting drawings, such as *draw how your parents see you, then draw how you see yourself,* prompts adolescents to imagine others' viewpoints, while satisfying their typical dichotomous view of the world. These approaches may soften the client's refusal to see the point of treatment.

A humanistic style in the therapist will be effective with most adolescents. Its reliance on therapist nonjudgmentalism (unconditional positive regard), empathy, and genuineness support the adolescent, rather than provoking defensiveness and an adversarial relationship. It can be assumed that an adolescent presenting for SAT has already encountered plenty of confrontational experiences with authority, and been given messages regarding "conditions of worth." If the art therapist joins this chorus, it is unlikely that the therapeutic relationship will become established, although the teen may still become involved with the art making.

Adolescents act out; they challenge adults to set limits at the same time that they refuse to abide by them. In so doing, they are working through dependency conflicts and seeking their own identity and values, which will provide the basis for future self-limits and mature behavior. Therapists should expect to be provoked, and try to refrain from overreacting. Challenges can become a teaching point when genuineness and empathy are felt and displayed.

A vignette from the literature exemplifies these issues. Riley (1999a) wrote of a time when it might be supposed that her unconditional positive regard was stretched beyond the limit. Six boys in their early teens came into the group room laughing over the fact that outside the clinic they had found a nest of baby birds and thrown them out into the street to be run over. Riley was outraged, but managed to locate her empathy and observe, "I suppose you have felt, at times, that life has tossed you out in the street to be run over" (p.218). However, this interpretative remark did not have the wished-for sobering effect on the boys, and in the face of their ongoing joking, she found that her anger was such that she could not honestly proceed. She told them that she was quite upset, that killing innocent life was abhorrent to her, and that they were dismissed from the session for the day. Although she does not say, it is likely that Riley's genuineness and transparency made a difference in the future relationship with these boys. If she had attempted to cover her disgust, it would have been to collude with their behavior. In addition, her verbalized correlation of the baby birds to their own experience of being "throwaways" signaled that she felt a deep compassion for them.

Individual work with adolescents

The importance of the initial alliance is paramount when working with adolescents in individual sessions. I used a carefully structured intake procedure for individual treatment in private practice that minimized the focus on substance abuse. Depending on the age of the client, I met first with the parent and teen together, explained that I would not in future be reporting back to the parent without discussing it first with the child, except in specified circumstances when I believed someone to be in danger, and then proceeded with the intake with the client alone.

In these first sessions, I found it important to be genuinely friendly and for the studio and art materials to be richly appealing. My verbal role was limited to imparting information about how therapy would proceed, asking careful questions, and listening. At the conclusion of the first session, I would ask the adolescent, "So, do you think this is something you will like to do?" If the answer was, "Well, I don't have any choice," I would empathize with that stuck place, suggest that we give it a try, and identify ways that the client *could* have choices within the treatment process.

Finding empathy for Suzanne

In Chapter 4, I discussed the value of informal assessment drawings as a way to bypass initial defensiveness. When I first encountered Suzanne, I had difficulty feeling any warmth or empathy for her, which was uncomfortable for me as well as being prohibitive for my preferred humanistic and MI/SOC therapeutic approach. Suzanne was a freshman at a community college who was struggling with cocaine and other drug use. Her referral source had told me she knew she needed to quit using, but was resistant to verbal therapy and in particular wouldn't talk about her family or her past, which was thought to involve sexual abuse. During her initial individual session with me, Suzanne presented as suspicious and marginally cooperative. After attempting initially to establish verbal rapport, I decided to ask her to make a Kinetic House-Tree-Person (K-H-T-P) drawing, which I presented as a simple drawing task that I sometimes used to get to know clients and their drawing style.

By the time she had finished drawing, it was apparent that this drawing prompt was all she needed to begin to communicate on a more honest level; in addition, my feelings toward her changed almost instantaneously (see Figure 8.5). In the drawing, shrubbery reminiscent of concertina wire guards a house with a prohibitively tiny door. Her wretched figure is huddled defensively under a streaming willow, and separated by the house from a fenced and padlocked side yard, which she described as the place of secrets where she did not want to go. I now had a deeply felt sense of this client's world and compassion regarding her dread of reviewing the past; I understood what lay behind her unattractive behaviors. The defensive ice was broken and we could proceed to begin working.

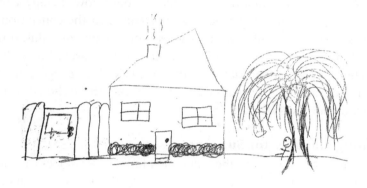

Figure 8.5: Suzanne's Kinetic House-Tree-Person (K-H-T-P) drawing

Adolescent group work

The benefits of group work for SAT in general has been discussed, with special emphasis on the therapeutic factors of universality and interpersonal learning. Benefits are similar for adolescent groups, although in my experience it can take longer to build cohesion than in adult groups. Perhaps more than in adult groups, the presence of a strong or charismatic member, whether they are a positive or negative influence, can sway the entire group identity. Attempts by the therapist to balance the group are not always successful. Sometimes groups react with a group mind; other times, an acting-out member is successfully ignored, but sometimes this requires the sacrifice of the therapeutic benefit of the group for that person.

Riley's story of experiencing anger toward her group of adolescent clients reminds me of an experience I had while working in an outpatient drug treatment setting. Because I was dually credentialed, the agency allowed me to make use of art therapy as I desired in both individual and small group modalities. I found art making to be indispensable in adolescent groups for its qualities of equalizing the players, containing stress, neutralizing the authority presence, and even of expressing positive feelings that were not allowed verbal expression by cynical adolescent personas. As is shown in this example, the art can also be used to communicate clearly when a client is bent on resistance.

Brandon's group

Brandon was an 18-year-old high school senior who had been referred by his parents, upon pressure from the school counselor, who cited Brandon's "bad attitude" and known drug usage that was interfering with his schoolwork. From what I could determine, his parents' true motivation was fear that he would not complete school and would continue to be a financial burden. Otherwise, there was a decided mixed message about the need to stop using drugs: Brandon's father was a member of a motorcycle gang whose activities included indiscriminant alcohol and drug use and whose philosophy advocated white supremacy. Brandon bragged to me about accompanying his father to rallies and campouts and their drug and alcohol use at those events. His parents expressed no interest in family therapy or in exploring their own substance use.

At the time of Brandon's first day in treatment, there were only two other clients in the adolescent program: Amy, a 16-year-old Caucasian, and Sherri, a 15-year-old African-American. I was horrified when Brandon introduced himself at the first group art therapy session by sharing specifics about his racist beliefs and gang affiliation. He did this in a practiced passive-aggressive manner that suggested he was utterly unaware that his speech might be threatening or irritating to others, or that if he was, it didn't matter because he had a right to do so. The two girls looked uncomfortable and kept their eyes down, saying nothing. The adolescent group room was situated in the basement of the treatment center with a small office in the corner. I asked the girls to make a check-in drawing and asked Brandon to come meet with me in the office for a few minutes. Once inside, I asked Brandon if he considered that what he had said might have been offensive. He said, "Oh, 'cause of *her*? I'm not talking about her. I wouldn't, like, hurt her or anything." He seemed very practiced at rationalizing his behavior.

I then inquired about the preliminary treatment goals that had been set up for Brandon with the intake counselor, although I was already familiar with them. He replied in a cynical tone that they were to "quit doing drugs" and "work on my bad attitude." I asked him what he thought would be entailed in addressing the latter goal, and he leaned back in his chair, eyed me directly, and replied with a sneer, "Lady, you only get me for six weeks! You can't *touch* my bad attitude." It was fortunate that my jaw actually dropped, thus delaying delivery of a comeback remark long enough for an empathetic thought to emerge in its place: that perhaps, growing up in a hate-group atmosphere, he had never had the opportunity to learn empathy or sensitivity to others. I decided I would let him win a round, at least in his own eyes, by not delivering a general lecture or ultimatum. Instead I reminded him of the group rule to respect others; explained that proclaiming beliefs that certain people were inherently inferior might seem disrespectful; and suggested that despite his avowed intent, his style might seem threatening to the younger girl, Sherri, who was sitting at the table with him.

We rejoined the group and I was glad to see the girls had been chatting. I told the group we would work individually to make drawings, and directed this version of the K-H-T-P: *draw a picture that has a house, a tree, and a person in it. You can add anything else you like*. I wanted to create a nonthreatening atmosphere, and felt this group was too new to process the effect of Brandon's prior discourse on the other group members. The fact that I had taken Brandon into the office after he spoke signaled to the girls that I would keep the space safe. I chose this directive because it had enough structure to keep the teens busy; it had not appeared to be personally confrontational; and it provided room for self-expression as well as unguarded projection.

Sherri's drawing was relatively unique in that it showed the inside of a house, or rather, as she explained, her family's apartment, with a tree visible outside a window, and herself seated at a table and drawing a picture of a another house. Her interpretation suggested she had created a place of safety for herself (the interior home setting) while creatively incorporating the task directions to include a house, tree, and person. She was obviously proud of her clever solution and was happy to share her drawing.

Amy had drawn a two-dimensional house and "lollipop" tree typical of Lowenfeld's schematic stage (Lowenfeld and Brittain 1987, first published 1947), although her person was drawn at a more advanced level. She depicted a girl with detailed clothing and carefully articulated makeup and hairstyle; this appeared to be an accurate self-image and to reflect healthy narcissism. She was also proud of her drawing. I was pleased that this task had been engaging and allowed the girls to share about themselves and to feel pride, without necessitating much verbal interaction with Brandon.

Brandon's drawing depicted a wild-eyed stick figure smoking a bong behind a tree, which both hid and animatedly protected the figure from a house/school/authority symbol. The girls did not seem to want to look at it, and Brandon did not want to describe it beyond saying, duh, he was smoking a bong. The girls were not prepared to give him feedback, and at any rate, the session time was over. I set an intention to build a fresh start with Brandon in our individual session the following morning, perhaps by creating a conjoint drawing (in the empty group room, on ample-sized paper!). However, he never returned to treatment. When our agency called his parents, they had capitulated to his decision to drop out of our outpatient program and refused to consider a referral for a residential setting, saying that he would "grow out of it" (see Schmanke 2016 for more about Brandon and his drawing).

The importance of the holding environment

Much adolescent acting-out may be interpreted as a response to overwhelming dependency needs that are in conflict with the desire to be grown and away from controlling or abusive authority. Groups with peers can provide a developmentally syntonic place to satisfy a need to be *held*, whereas an individual session with an adult therapist stirs up counter-dependency and resentment. The creation of a *holding environment* (see Winnicott 2005, first published 1971), particularly one with artistic play instead of verbal demands, meets the remedial developmental needs of adolescents who lacked these experiences in the home. The role of the therapist is to approximate the mirroring, approving caretaker who is present as a secure base for the child to explore the environment and practice new abilities. Therapists make groups a safe container by setting limits, encouraging mutual respect, and building a positive experience of activity and talk in a social setting.

Brandon's one experience of group treatment was not successful in the sense that his progression in treatment halted. But maybe at some point during that session with me and with his peers he had encountered the idea that a healthy group could be a safe place to experience a supportive holding environment, one where respect felt good. I hoped that sometime in the future Brandon would find his way to another positive peer group, whether in school, treatment, or a self-help setting, where he could experience the validation and assistance it could provide.

9

Families in Crisis and in Recovery

This chapter begins with an overview of issues in family systems where substance abuse is or has been present. Even for therapists who never plan to work with families or couples, it is important to understand these concepts, because they are likely to describe the original family system of clients with SUD. Psychoeducation about the issues in this chapter is often incorporated into addiction treatment, to enable self-understanding as well as to address or prevent ongoing family problems. The chapter goes on to discuss current approaches to family work in the substance abuse field as well as pertinent art therapy approaches, and concludes with a case example of art therapy with a family whose presenting problem initially obscured the presence of generational issues.

Family theory pertaining to addictions

In the 1980s and early 1990s, public awareness of codependency and so-called dysfunctional family roles and dynamics was at a height. This was due in large part to research on substance-abusing families and writing for the popular press by professionals such as psychologist Janet Woititz, social worker Claudia Black, and family therapist Sharon Wegscheider-Cruse, a protégé of family therapy pioneer Virginia Satir, who began to look specifically at alcoholic families and to identify their unique dynamics and family roles. Other popular authors and speakers achieved celebrity status for addressing healing for partners and family members, including John Bradshaw (*Healing the Shame that Binds You*, 1988) and Melody Beattie (*Codependent No More*, 1986).

Although overly broad definitions of the term *codependent* generated ridicule, the consciousness-raising of this era led to public realization that the partners, children, and other family members of substance abusers developed problematic coping behaviors of their own. Further, it was seen that without intervention, these personal dynamics continued even if the addicted person recovered, and even into the next generation. Research on children of alcoholics revealed that as adults, a majority developed substance abuse problems themselves and/or partnered with people with addictions, and thus repeated the family pattern (McCollum and Trepper 2001). The term *dysfunctional family*, once used to describe such patterns, is now considered derogatory in addition to being inaccurate. These families may *function* quite well, in that they are able to maintain relative homeostasis, but this is achieved in unhealthy ways that perpetuate the root problem.

Use of a family systems approach involves looking at addiction as a problem within a family system, rather than looking at a disease in a particular person. Systems therapy can peaceably coexist with other SAT approaches, but it entails different goals, such as identifying family strengths and solutions. It also focuses on changing the roles and rules that the families have developed in an attempt to control the addict's behavior.

Family rules, dynamics, and roles

Family rules

Foremost among the unspoken rules in these family systems is the triad articulated by Black (1981) as *don't talk, don't trust, don't feel*.

- *Don't talk:* Family members maintain the illusion both within the system and to the outside world that they are a "normal" family. Children understand the implicit direction not to remark on the inconsistent behaviors of the addict. Because the effects of the substance use are usually obvious to the children, the refusal of the codependent parent to affirm what is happening can lead them to doubt their own interpretations of reality. This contributes to the common feeling, even in adulthood, that they have to guess at what normal is (Woititz 1990, first published 1983).

- *Don't trust:* Family members learn not to trust the person with addiction issues (PWAI), as they are bound to be betrayed or disappointed. This applies to both implied and explicit responsibilities, including attendance at special events, financial contributions, or promises of change. The PWAI is also likely to be unpredictable in mood and behavior, with the result that family members feel that they are continually walking on eggshells and unable to trust in any kind of predictable daily life.

- *Don't feel:* Family members' feelings are discounted; any natural responses to the family predicament or events, including anger, resentment, bitterness, shame, disappointment, and grief, must be suppressed. A corollary to this rule is that only the PWAI is allowed to express negative feelings, which might range from chemically augmented rage to maudlin self-pity.

The dynamics of codependency

Unhealthy behaviors beget unhealthy responses, which may then continue in a vicious cycle and result in rigid roles or personas. The term *codependent* originated in reference to the partner of a substance-dependent person, who becomes *dependent* on that person, specifically on the dynamic created by the substance abuse. In other words, the codependent becomes obsessed with the addict and addict's behaviors in a manner that echoes the drug addictive behavior. Codependents may attempt to control an addict by begging, bargaining, nagging, threatening, hiding the drug, joining in use, or other means. They may take the role of the family *martyr* wherein they continually remind the others of their sacrifice in putting up with the addict. Their unpleasant behaviors are generally ineffectual, except to give the addict another excuse to use.

Another role commonly identified in the partner of an addict is the *enabler*. A codependent partner is said to *enable* the partner's addiction by behaviors such as making excuses to others for drug-related absences from work or social functions, and taking care of situations, from wrecked cars to failed parenting situations with children. When an enabling wife literally cleans up her drunken husband and puts him to bed, he is spared the discomfort of waking on the floor in his own urine or vomit; the children are spared the sight of their father in such a state; and her own wrecked self-esteem is assuaged by martyrdom. The pattern of enabling serves to avert crises and maintains family stability or homeostasis; however, it ultimately harms the entire family, and protects the addict from natural consequences that might otherwise lead to seeking treatment.

Enabling behavior is usually most entrenched in the spouse or intimate companion of an addict, although it may also be performed by children or others in the addict's life. When families seek treatment, the child in the scapegoat role (more below) is often the first to speak openly or complain about the unfairness of enabling behavior. This can be an opportunity to guide discussion of how the family might start a new rule that everyone is responsible in dealing with the consequences of their own actions, with appropriate adjustments for the person's age. When the addicted family member is still using, disruption of enabling is best addressed as an early goal.

The word *enabling* generally has a positive connotation, as it is used in the subtitle of this book. It is important to educate family members at any stage of treatment that when the term *enabling* is used specifically in reference to codependent behavior, it is limited to this concept of enabling the negative (addictive) behavior. This concept of enabling does not apply to helping someone who is in *recovery*. I make this point because I have had parents tell me they would like to help their grown child who is in recovery, but "we don't want to enable him." Enabling *recovery* is a positive goal for family members; it provides the support needed for the person to gain a firm footing in sobriety, and indicates caring, forgiveness, and confidence in the person's ability to change. In fact, it can make a significant difference in the person's prognosis. Ironically, many families who financially support an actively addicted member for years will snap the wallet closed when the person finally enters recovery and has legitimate need of help. The collapse of the dysfunctional dynamic, caused by the person entering recovery, may create such a passive-aggressive response. Regardless, it is the right of families to draw the line at further assistance, especially if they are not confident of the person's continued sobriety. This may also reflect the family's newfound ability to be assertive with regard to boundaries and behaviors. The point in therapy is to make these issues transparent.

Individuals with codependency issues who are ready to change, whether or not the PWAI is entering recovery, will benefit from participation in self-help groups such as Al-Anon, Nar-Anon, or Adult Children of Alcoholics, or by seeking individual or group therapy. The challenges of working with codependency are similar to working with addiction. In cases where an intimate partner of an addict appears to be truly addicted to that person or dynamic, they may even suffer physical withdrawal symptoms when attempting to detach and strengthen boundaries. Without self-help support or treatment, codependents are likely to remain entrenched in a relationship with a chronically using or relapsing partner—or to recreate the pattern with a new partner, perhaps creating more families with the unhealthy dynamic.

Roles typical of children

Children's roles in an unhealthy family system are not about choice, although a role may feel comfortable to the child because it seems to be the best way to cope and is reinforced by the parents. Because the family focus is on maintaining homeostasis in the face of the addictive chaos, children have little freedom to drop roles or behaviors or to explore new ones.

Table 9.1 identifies typical children's roles in an alcoholic family system, as described in the work of Wegscheider-Cruse (1991, first published 1976), whose work grew from her application of Satir's roles theory specifically to families with an alcoholic parent, and later to families with comparable dynamics. This model and others (e.g., Black 1981) are still widely in use for psychoeducation and therapeutic applications in SAT.

Table 9.1 Roles typical of children in a family with parental substance abuse

Role name	Family hero	Scapegoat	Lost child	Mascot
Typical sibling order	Often the oldest child, especially if female	May be second child, often male	Often the third or middle child	Often the youngest child
School functioning	Makes good grades, teacher's pet; many extracurricular activities; a leader	Gets in trouble, fails, or is truant; may appear not to care; is disorganized	Quiet, shy, tends to go unnoticed by teachers and peers	Class clown; distractible and distracting; may be diagnosed with ADHD
External identity	Organized; serious, adult-like, seldom plays; relatives have high expectations and rely on; helpful at home, takes on adult family roles; acts as mother to siblings, confidante to one or both parents; may make family decisions	May originally try to do as well as the hero but fails or gives up; family doesn't show pride or compares unfavorably to hero; blamed for things for which not responsible; may withdraw, rebel, or indulge in acting-out behaviors	Loner; may spend most time alone in activities like reading, TV, video games; tries not to be a bother; strong attachment to animals, toys, or tech; usually no close friends	Happy-go-lucky, energetic, often charming; may exaggerate own dependency needs so family can regard as in need of protection or assistance; provides family with a distraction at tense moments
Internal characteristics	Never feels good enough, since despite unceasing efforts to be perfect, the family dysfunction is not affected; stressed and afraid of breaking down and causing disaster; feels guilty, scared, lonely	Feels left out in the family; needs and longs for normal attention but can't ask for it; often is the family member least in denial of the real problem; feels like a misfit in life; angry, lonely, guilty, hurt	Feels "different," feels like an outsider who is observing life; low self-worth; feels forgotten; no sense of goals or direction; may experience panic or deep anxiety	Knows something is wrong but no one else acknowledges it to them; may doubt own sanity; fearful, anxious, confused; power and relief lie in making others laugh or seem happy
Family need addressed	Makes family look good to the outside world; provides esteem and assurance that the parents are good people	Provides a scapegoat for blaming specific situations and an overall problem focus, which supports denial of the real problem	Does not stress the family system emotionally; provides a drain for the drama; low maintenance	Provides humor; allows the family a semblance at properly nurturing a child ("the baby of the family")

Content adapted from Wegscheider-Cruse (1991)

Children may occupy more than one role at once, or may unconsciously shift from one role to another in response to the changing needs of the family. For example, when a hero child grows up and moves away, the lost child may need to step up to the role of proving to the outside world that the family is good. Similarly, a mascot may begin to act out in a blameworthy rather than charming manner, to replace the function of a scapegoat who has left the family.

Adult children

The formal term "adult children of alcoholics" (ACOAs or ACAs) is often shortened to *adult children* to reference adults whose childhood was spent in a family with an addiction dynamic. Broadly speaking, adult children tend to have problems in adulthood that echo their childhood experience (Wegscheider-Cruse 1989, first published 1981; Woititz 1990). The overachieving hero child may become an over-controlling workaholic who has difficulty relaxing and enjoying social situations or intimate relationships. Substance addiction may be successfully hidden from the outside world. Career success may be achieved, but it is not experienced internally as success, just as earlier markers of success could never cure the parental addiction.

The scapegoat's frustration, resentment, and anger may carry over into adult acting-out, often including substance abuse, with relational or legal consequences. The poor self-esteem internalized with this role may be masked by bravado or grandiosity.

The lost child continues to attempt to feel secure by maintaining invisibility, which leads to isolation, depression, and feelings of being unwanted. Children in this role may become adults who prefer to let others manage their lives; they often partner with PWAI.

The mascot, who uses charm to make others happy and support their denial of anything wrong, will continue to feel most comfortable when making others laugh or feel better. Adults may be drawn to careers in the performing arts or to helping careers such as counseling, teaching, or nursing, but without therapy, they may continue to experience inner sadness, confusion, or anxiety.

Standard treatment approaches for families with substance abuse issues

Although they share many common characteristics, families with substance-abusing members are far from a homogenous population. Treatment should be individualized according to the dominant presenting problem, as articulated by the family; providers should explain that goals and approaches may evolve over time. The following are examples of typical goals from various stages of recovery (not necessarily in order):

- assess or treat the identified patient (often a child who is acting out and experimenting with drugs, when the deeper problem lies with a parental addiction)
- persuade the substance-abusing person to get into treatment
- learn to properly support a family member in recovery while maintaining new roles and boundaries, and
- work on family recovery from codependent behaviors and roles when a substance-using member is no longer living with the family.

Depending on the presenting problem, goals, and family resources, any one or combination of the following methods may be beneficial for instigating or providing treatment.

Self-help groups

Al-Anon was founded officially in 1951 by Lois Wilson, wife of AA co-founder Bill Wilson, who recognized that an "illness" was contracted by spouses of still-using and recovering alcoholics, and that they needed to have their own support and recovery fellowship. Sharing in Al-Anon meetings focuses on the self and the effect of alcoholism on one's own life and behaviors, rather than on the alcoholic. Alateen provides similar groups for teenagers, which are facilitated by Al-Anon members who have completed a certification process. Nar-Anon and Narateen are corresponding groups affiliated with Narcotics Anonymous (NA) for friends and family of problem drug users. Adult Children of Alcoholics is another self-help group for those whose problematic behaviors have developed as a response to living with an alcoholic parent; again, the focus is on personal change, not on blame or attempting to change others (Stevens and Smith 2013).

Intervention

V. Johnson (1986) was an early substance abuse counseling theorist and one of the first to promote the idea that an alcoholic didn't need to "hit bottom" (in the sense of losing health, job, or family) to benefit from treatment. Johnson originated a structured process known as family intervention, which consisted of a surprise meeting wherein a substance abuser is confronted by family members, employers, or friends, along with a substance abuse counselor. The various participants provide the addict with examples of their addiction-related behavior that harmed their relationships or led to other undesirous consequences. The substance abuser is then offered an immediate referral to treatment (typically, tentative arrangements have already been made); participants specify the consequences of refusal (the addict will lose their job, must move out of the home, etc.).

Although this approach has been popularized on reality TV, many in the field now view the Johnson-style intervention as a holdover of the confrontational approach to SAT, which has generally been supplanted by more motivational-style approaches. However, confrontational-style interventions are still in use, and some research has indicated their effectiveness compared to other types of referral to treatment (Loneck, Garrett, and Banks 1996). The bottom line for the persistence of this approach may be that a one-time confrontation done in the safety of a counselor's presence has understandable appeal for long-suffering family members. Although a responsible intervention counselor would not instill this idea during preparation, partners or families may fantasize about a wonderful cathartic experience, after which the substance abuser will see the light, or at least be removed from them for a time to attend residential treatment.

Embedded family groups

Many treatment programs provide family sessions that consist of psychoeducational groups or brief multifamily treatment interventions. The primary goal is to support the addict's recovery by providing information about the nature of addiction and how the family can best help the person avoid relapse. General information about family rules, roles, and dynamics may also be provided, along with referrals to self-help groups for family members. At some agencies, multifamily therapy may be available.

Combined approaches

A motivational model known as Community Reinforcement and Family Training (CRAFT) (Meyers *et al.* 1999) is representative of newer "combined" approaches for families. The goal of getting the substance abuser into treatment, or into a reduced-harm level of use, is combined with the goal of promoting healthier behaviors and stress reduction in the entire family. Family members learn to apply principles of behavior modification to influence the problem user to seek treatment. Healthy behaviors are rewarded by positive engagement, and substance-using times are ignored; CRAFT teaches families that addicts should not be protected from the natural consequences of their behaviors. This approach has been shown to be significantly more effective in influencing treatment-resistant people to seek treatment than confrontational-style interventions (Meyers *et al.* 1999), in addition to providing the benefits of improved relational skills and reduced stress in family members.

Family art therapy with addiction issues

The value of art therapy for family therapy in general has been well articulated in the work of many authors over the years. Art therapists working with families for whom substance abuse is a particular issue need to balance knowledge and skills in the three areas of family therapy, art therapy, and substance abuse treatment.

The therapist may find it helpful to practice principles of Motivational Interviewing (MI) in order to engage a substance-abusing family member. It is likely that a person who is still using will not participate on a deep level during family sessions, and may not even attend regularly. When a still-using member is engaged in a family session, but not with the goal of sobriety, the therapist will want to *roll with resistance* and acknowledge the client's feelings of ambiguity toward further treatment. The therapist may consider providing a psychoeducational session with the addict's partner or family to inform them about this therapeutic approach.

An awareness of the concept of the identified patient is important. Even when a parent has an active addiction, the child in the scapegoat role is often the identified client or symptom-bearer who gets the family into treatment. It may be necessary to go along with this interpretation of the family problem until the therapeutic relationship is established; however, if the spotlight continues to fall on the scapegoat, they are unlikely to continue to attend or to be cooperative (Minuchin 1993). The therapist must maintain awareness that the scapegoat is in an impossible position: the unspoken mandate to the child is to maintain the scapegoat identity in order to ensure the family homeostasis, while the overt mandate is to comply with therapy to change that very identity. One way to move this process forward is with the *draw your problem* directive. Just as this task provides a wealth of information when working with an individual in SAT, asking each family member to *draw the family's problem* will provide an insight into each individual's perspective and provoke meaningful discussion.

Art products often serve to communicate what is known but has not been verbalized due to the *don't talk* rule. Family members who would not otherwise dare to implicate another family member or reveal personal negative emotions may communicate those messages in the art, either overtly or metaphorically. In order to encourage such self-disclosure, the art therapist may decide to stipulate that family members are not required to talk about their art products unless they wish. While on the surface this may seem to mirror the unhealthy *don't talk* rule, it acknowledges the power of the art to communicate without words while providing a feeling of safety.

Techniques using family photographs can move therapy forward quickly for families, as well as for individuals who are reexamining the role of childhood experience in their adult issues. PhotoTherapy founder Judy Weiser (1999, first published 1993) identified two particular values of these techniques: helping to uncover and process the less-conscious aspects of abuse experience in a client's past, and providing perspective for people facing crises including personal problems. Art therapists working with people from dysfunctional families can design activities using copies of family photographs to reflect upon, or experiment with changes to, family roles or dynamics. In the example shown in Figure 9.1, manipulation and collaging of a family photo originally taken by the alcoholic family member allowed exploration of the theme of "looking-good kids" who present an image of the family's respectability to the community, but who are themselves guessing at what is normal (Black 1981).

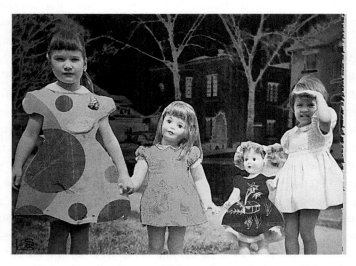

Figure 9.1: Photo collage: "Looking-good kids, guessing at what's normal" (see color plate)

Landgarten (1987) warned art therapists to contemplate the timing and therapeutic value of activities that can elicit strong emotions or bring out family secrets. Understanding the readiness of each family member is an important consideration. Paying attention to media quality is one way to control response; drier media support intellectual defenses, while less controllable media may enable greater risk-taking, emotional expression, or regression. At some point, families realize that taking risks in art therapy sessions is a practice step for taking similar risks at home. They can be helped to understand that the rigid rules and defenses they have acquired are normal, but ultimately unhealthy, coping mechanisms.

Family art productions are often rich with symbolic meaning that may be quite apparent to the art therapist, but it is important that the therapist not interpret imagery for the clients, particularly in the early stages. Denial can be quite powerful, and denial related to addictions can be so extreme that it appears ridiculous to observers. Even well-trained therapists will think, "How can they not see what their addiction is doing to the family?!" Similarly, imagery with meaning that would be blatantly obvious to anyone else may not be understood by family members. If the art therapist interprets, or suggests interpretations too soon, consequences may include feelings of insult, increased defensiveness, or even termination of treatment. Often, the person in the scapegoat role will be the first to become aware of metaphors that reveal issues behind denial and will break the *don't talk* rule.

Educating clients about typical addiction family dynamics helps families realize they're not unique. The therapist can also educate about denial and other ego defenses, and point out imagery that conveys double messages, such as a person appearing to smile and cry simultaneously. A participant who draws such an image may be totally unaware of the discrepancy, which suggests the ego defense of isolation of affect. In the case of an addicted family member, the smiling face with tears may reflect internal feelings of guilt or despair, which are hidden by the smile of bravado or denial.

Reaction formation, another ego defense that often accompanies denial, is also frequently in evidence. In one session, the wife of a violent alcoholic drew the house in a Kinetic House-Tree-Person (K-H-T-P) task very neatly, with a little picket fence and window boxes filled with flowers. This session became quite powerful when the husband grew aware of the defensive nature of her image, and became tearful looking at the drawing. He pointed at one of her perfect fantasy windows and explained that in reality he had broken that window in a drunken rage. His wife had communicated wordlessly and even unconsciously, but so poignantly that he gained insight and was moved to share his own feelings of guilt and sorrow at failing her. This example also demonstrates the ability of the concrete evidence of the art to confront resistance and denial, while allowing the art therapist to be perceived as being on the family's side as a participant observer.

Simple art directives that recall Satir's family sculpting techniques (McCollum and Trepper 2001) can be used to explore the family members' relationships in a nonthreatening manner. For example, each family member might be asked to create a self symbol with clay; all are then asked to place them in appropriate relation to each other. The therapist silently observes who goes first and the relative placement of images, as well as participants' description of their representations. Callaghan (1993) provided a similar directive using collage images. Further, each member may be given the opportunity to rearrange the images as they would like to have them. This serves to provide further input about structural changes that might improve flexibility in family functioning. The art therapist may ask the family members to reflect upon the process, and to identify dominant or passive members, as well as any subgroups.

When working with the Wilson family, I used elements of a structural approach, which requires the therapist to partner as an active investigator into family functioning. A primary methodology is to identify and rebalance enmeshed or disengaged subsystems, and to allow expansion of role identities (Minuchin 1993). This approach is well suited to help codependent family members recognize inaccurate definitions of family problems, adjust over-functioning behaviors, and create healthier boundaries with each other. Hoshino (2008) pointed out that art therapy is a good fit with the structural family approach, since art making levels the playing field to enable role balancing. Disempowered or timid family members have an equal say when it comes to art products, and members who are more aggressive or who favor verbally expressed defense mechanisms are required to be quiet and express themselves nonverbally.

The Wilson family

Parents of children with substance use problems who are referred for family therapy usually anticipate being viewed as responsible for the child's problems. It is important to educate parents about the purpose of family therapy, which is not to uncover addiction etiology, but to look at how the family system may contribute to the maintenance of family problems. The etiology of the addiction itself is portrayed as a complicated biopsychosocial (BPS) issue that is beyond the scope of family treatment. Family art therapy may be described as less stressful or more playful than verbal family therapy. These factors were all relevant in the case of the Wilsons, whose need for family therapy was accurately perceived by the addictions counselor who was already working individually with their daughter.

Background

The Wilsons agreed to come to family art therapy at the SAT clinic where they had sought help for their teenage daughter, Paige, who had been using alcohol and marijuana. Paige was attending individual outpatient sessions with the adolescent addictions counselor, who believed her substance use had been light and that she had significant personal strengths, but suspected systemic issues and recommended family therapy. Paige's brother Danny, age 13, mother, Bethany, and stepfather of two years, Stan, would attend the sessions. Bethany's ex-husband, who was the children's father, was reported to be in a severe chronic stage of alcohol abuse and was not currently involved with the family or the therapy.

Paige was an attractive high-school senior who had fallen in love with Blaine, a 21-year-old restaurant worker who was on probation for a misdemeanor marijuana offense. Paige and Blaine were upfront about the fact that both used alcohol (Blaine was old enough to do so legally); Bethany suspected that they used marijuana and possibly other drugs. Two months prior, the pair had run off together for two days, but had returned when Paige wanted to get back to school. Bethany was extremely anxious over her daughter's relationship with Blaine, which had eclipsed her own formerly close relationship with her daughter. Since Paige's runaway escapade, Bethany had responded with extreme rules and curfews, and then struggled with her own desire to enforce them in the face of the predictable dramatic repercussions. Initially, Stan complied with the extreme limit-setting, although he advocated taking a more hands-off approach to parenting older teens. He insinuated that Bethany's overreaction to Paige's behaviors was driving her further away. I knew from the agency intake report that Bethany's parents had experienced severe problems with alcohol during her own childhood and adolescence. She had continued the family pattern when she married the children's father, who even at that time had an obvious alcohol problem.

Danny was described by his mother as a good boy who had a mild learning disability. Stan reported that Danny loved physical activities and being outside; it appeared that the stepfather was providing healthy parenting for the boy, perhaps being more involved with him than Bethany.

My intention in working with this family was to help them gain perspective on their own behaviors, and to learn about the lasting dynamics for families touched by addiction, even when an addicted person is no longer present. A structural lens would help me identify subsystems that required rebalancing. The intake report indicated that this family had above-average resources and strengths, and it appeared that they were going through a relatively normal developmental crisis. I believed that an enlarged perspective would help explain current problems, and help them to feel more normal, less panicky, and better able to rely on their own strengths to deal with problems. However, it was important to align with each family member's presentation of the issues at the beginning of therapy. I couldn't make either Paige or her mother "wrong," although I wanted to soften the focus on Paige's behaviors, as I believed they were only a symptom of the family issues. I suspected that Bethany was continuing in a typical untreated ACA behavior of struggling to stave off anxiety by controlling all around her. Rebalancing this family would involve helping her identify and vacate these codependent responses, by which she could help release Paige from her combined hero/scapegoat and Danny from his lost child/mascot roles. I planned to suggest that since the "identified patient" of the family was already doing well in individual drug treatment, in the family art therapy sessions we could work on issues other than Paige's substance use.

Initial art therapy session

For the initial session, my primary goal was to align with the family and help them relax, trust me, and feel good about family art therapy. This objective needs to be in any family therapist's awareness when starting out, but perhaps particularly with any family experiencing addiction or past addiction. The belief that the substance abuser is the only one who needs therapy is very strong. It is difficult to engage all members so that they attend consistently, or even want to return for a second session. A secondary goal for myself in the first session was to learn about the family as individuals and observe their family dynamics *in vivo*.

The first family art task was a nonthreatening stimulus drawing with a pre-drawn prompt of a blank billboard, with the directive *create a billboard about you*. Colored pencils were offered to allow for a feeling of control, yet to require use of color. Paige seemed to enjoy the task, and made full use of the colored pencils to shade her lettering and symbols artistically. She used an in-vogue lettering style to write her initials, those of her high school, and Blaine's nickname, and included emblems of interest such as her phone, hearts, her favorite earrings, a comb and scissors for her interest in pursuing cosmetology, a playful leaping dolphin, a schematic sun in the corner of the billboard, and her favorite teddy bear from childhood. Although these happy, healthy elements could have been drawn intentionally to mislead the authority figures in the room, Paige's forthright and ingenuous style supported a face-value interpretation of this typical high-school girl's symbol drawing.

Stepfather Stan, along with Paige, seemed to enjoy the activity, and depicted a large smiling sun, as well as carefully drawn, colored, and labeled symbols for his job, which involved interfacing with the public, and his favorite sports and hobbies. In addition he wrote a list of his good qualities: "Extreme worker; Good at all sports; Not many worries; Fun to be with or around; Loves to make people happy when working!!!" Stan's gregarious and perhaps also grandiose personality was thus revealed. Creating this task alongside the children seemed to allow him to express himself in a childlike manner, and he engaged happily as if it were a family fun event he had planned himself.

Paige's brother Danny used orange and brown pencils exclusively to depict a stick figure on a skateboard, a video game controller, and a basketball backboard and hoop with a stick figure wearing a ball cap making a slam dunk. He had written his first and last name, as well as the words "Running," "Skateboarding," and "Snowboarding," properly spelled. Altogether, the drawing was appropriate for a boy his age.

Bethany alone appeared to be daunted by the directive and hesitated for several minutes as she tried to decide what to draw. She stalled by making comments about her lack of artistic ability and repeated, "I don't know what to put." It was not until Stan suggested she depict bowling (also one of his hobbies; he had drawn a bowling pin labeled "300," a perfect score) that she began to draw. After several minutes of hesitant drawing, she noticed her daughter's image of her toy bear, and stated happily that it gave her the idea to include the Mickey Mouse cap she had treasured as a child. It was later noted that this behavior of admiring or "copying" something of her daughter's had echoes in the family dynamic.

Notable in Bethany's drawing was an overall lack of color and stark drawing style. She had made a wood-brown bowling lane that stretched at an angle across the billboard. The sketchy quality of the gray-colored gutters on either side of the lane suggested anxiety, perhaps associated with the danger of the family metaphorically going into the gutter, or the confining generational path in her family history being defined by "gutter drunks." I could also imagine her alcoholic ex-husband being in the gutter on the one side and Paige's supposed drug-culture boyfriend on the other, as Bethany, symbolized as her favorite bowling ball, attempted to navigate safe passage. The bowling pins were not in view, although the ball was in progress down the lane. This seemed to represent a problem that could not be approached with confidence; the target was unknown. The three black circles identified as a Mickey Mouse emblem could have reflected the triad of herself and her two children; as she had with the gutters, she spent much time enhancing and darkening these three shapes with the black colored pencil. This symbol might also tie in to her awareness of family newcomer Stan's view of the family drama as unnecessary "Mickey Mouse stuff."

I kept my feelings about the drawings to myself, and asked the family to relate fun stories about each other suggested by the items in the billboards, if this could be done respectfully in my presence. I praised them when they were able to comply, and pointed out the strengths I observed: a strong family identity, true caring for each other, and behaviors of mutual respect, which were revealed both during the drawing session and in the sharing of stories. I explained that this session was important to establish perspective about the good things going on for their family, and also to show them that art therapy was a great way to work together.

Shifting of the identified patient

During a subsequent session when Danny was absent, the family agreed that Bethany's anxiety and paranoia (her own descriptor) over Paige's life was a major, wearying influence on family life. Stan had begun to challenge what he saw as Bethany's endless worrying and over-involvement with her daughter. As a result, Paige found herself attempting the reality-bending task of trying to make peace between parents who were arguing over how to respond to her own behaviors. When Paige was able to articulate some of this through a *draw how your parents see you / draw how you see yourself* drawing, Bethany seemed crushed. She stated that she had been wondering if some of her anxiety was linked to the fact that when she was younger, she had experienced many negative events tied to family and intimate relationships and substance abuse; however, she believed that Paige was a stronger, healthier person than she had been, so she wasn't sure that made sense.

Bethany and Paige attended the family art therapy session alone the next week, which allowed us to focus on the family subsystem that held the outstanding presenting issues. Using one large piece of poster board to represent the sea, I asked each to draw a "fantasy deserted island" including a dream home and whatever geographical or other features they would love to have in their ideal environment. Bethany seemed much more relaxed about drawing this time, and drew an unusual and beautiful home that was nestled in a forest that took up her entire island. Paige's house was a pink mansion bounded on two sides by being placed in the corner of the paper. On the other two sides, the house was bounded by a colorful garden and a garden wall that extended completely around its perimeter. When the pair appeared to be nearly done drawing, I asked if they would be able to visit each other from these very separate islands. Paige looked up and grinned as if having thought of this already, and immediately began to draw a large boat dock and a sailboat in which to go see her mother. Bethany followed her lead, drawing her own dock that was positioned to make Paige's boat trip the shortest possible.

In discussing their lovely homes, each revealed a longing for peace and beauty. Both these clients seemed ready for interpretive insight, and it was natural to segue to a discussion of their mutual wish for less drama at home. I pondered aloud whether maybe even a mutual desire for firmer boundaries between them was revealed by the encasement of their homes in physical features such as Bethany's dense forest and Paige's wall and paper-siding. We then talked about how a desire for self-time and strengthened boundaries could coexist with being able to communicate and "visit" each other. They seemed relieved that these wishes could be articulated.

Believing that they were ready for further self-examination, I remarked that in some ways, the pair seemed more like sisters than mother and daughter. I recalled that when I had asked them to compare and contrast themselves at the beginning of the session, they had both brightened and made reference to how much they were alike. They were obviously close, but Paige often seemed more mature and self-possessed; she evinced motherly concern over Bethany's struggles with anxiety. On the other hand, Bethany was feeling too overwhelmed to serve as a stable motherly guide and resource as Paige managed typical issues of late adolescence such as intimate relationships, substance use, and career planning. Bethany's anxiety was looking like the presenting problem for this family. Although ostensibly the anxiety was due to Paige's behaviors, it appeared that Bethany's earlier inkling was correct, and that it had other, more historical, roots.

I shared with the pair that I believed the strength of their relationship was a plus, although the role emphasis might be off-balance; I wondered aloud if this could lead to guilt or resentment. They agreed and were even forthcoming with verbal examples of Paige mothering Bethany. In concluding our session, I complimented them for their support of each other, and averred that they appeared to have turned a corner in their relationship.

Summary

These three strong initial sessions, despite the attrition in family member attendance, established trust and were a solid basis for further explorations. It came to light that Bethany had met her alcoholic husband at the same age that Paige was currently, which led to deeper insight for Bethany about her extreme anxiety that Paige's future would be ruined by her relationship with Blaine. Although the latter relationship did deserve attention, the family came to agree that Bethany's untreated issues from childhood in an alcoholic family and subsequent codependency issues in her first marriage were interfering with her ability to be her best self for Paige and Danny, and a relaxed partner with Stan. Bethany agreed to attend individual therapy as Paige continued with her individual counselor. The family met again for a follow-up art therapy session several weeks later, and even appeared glad to be with each other, reporting positive changes at home. They enjoyed creating a family forest (see Appendix A), which reinforced their individual strengths as well as demonstrating their cohesiveness.

Families often present for therapy with the scapegoat child as the identified client, whereas it is actually a parent's substance use that is at the root of the family dysfunction. In this case, a child's substance misuse was the red herring for a parent's untreated codependency issues that resulted from an addictive family history. Imagery and art therapy processing that occurred in the first few sessions led to speedy clarification of this family's problems, which in turn led to appropriate shifts in approach and successful treatment.

Appendix A
Selected Techniques and Activities

This appendix provides details for a few of the activities referenced previously in the book. Over the years, art therapists have derided so-called cookbook directives of the type that may be found in manualized approaches to substance abuse treatment (SAT). Conger (1988) was one of the first art therapists to publish about a creative yet "specific objectives approach" (p.34) for art therapy. By matching her suicidal adolescent clients' individual profiles and needs to specific goals, and thus to objectives tied to art directives, a clear picture of the effectiveness of the art therapy could be provided to treatment stakeholders in managed care settings.

Formulating art therapy themes in a lesson plan format may make them more palatable to drug treatment administrators concerned with demonstrating outcomes in documentation. Art therapists who take this approach need to educate treatment teams about the need for specific training in art therapy, which keeps implementation of these plans safe and relevant for each individual. Art therapists must be continually aware of individual and group needs, respond extemporaneously, and alter or substitute activities when it is indicated. Even art therapists who work with well-established directives must be wary not to fall into rote delivery of these activities.

Biopsychosocial-spiritual psychoeducational art activity ("BPSS pie") (Chapter 2)

Creating psychoeducational handouts to accompany art directives is another good way to build art therapy into a curriculum and reinforce and personalize learning. For the BPSS pie activity, the script consists of directions given by the group art therapist, who then leads discussion on the separate aspects as given in the handout. It is often difficult for participants to retain newly learned information when trying to conceptualize their art product, so it is helpful to provide a hard copy for reference as they work. If time allows, it can be beneficial to make three pies, one for the origins/etiology of their addiction; another for its current presentation; and a third one representing considerations for treatment, both proactive behaviors as well as relapse avoidance tactics.

Materials:

- 9" × 12" white paper with a predrawn circle using a compass set for a 7" diameter circle. This can be placed toward the top of the page, so as to allow room below the circle for participants to make a legend.
- Additional lined paper and pencils.
- Colored pencils, markers, and/or oil pastels.

Script:

In this activity, you will create a personalized, artistic version of a *pie chart* (a chart that depicts the parts of something in their relative sizes as slices of a pie). Your pie will represent the biopsychosocial-spiritual (BPSS) aspects of your addiction, so it will most likely have four slices. (If desired, describe making three charts, one about the *etiology* or contributing causes, another about the *current characteristics* of the problem, and the last about what *recovery* will involve.)

I'll start by explaining about the BPSS aspects, and you can use the lined paper to jot ideas for the slices of your pie. Feel free to ask questions as we go. When we're done talking, start creating your pie chart by using a pencil to draw lines dividing your circle into appropriately sized slices for each component: bio, psycho, social, and spiritual.

The relative sizes will be different for everyone. For example, if someone started using heroin for pain relief after their Vicodin prescription ran out, and they are only using heroin because it is too awful to go into withdrawal, the "bio" slice of their pie would be the biggest. On the other hand, if someone is highly involved with the club scene, and doesn't really drink or use except when they go out to a club, their "social" piece of the pie would be the biggest. But even in clear-cut cases like these, people will probably have at least a little slice of each of the four aspects. Think carefully about all your possibilities and make notes as I talk, and you will also receive a handout of the same material to review. Once you've identified your personal characteristics with regard to each of the four categories, decide on the relative sizes of your four pie pieces and divide your circle accordingly. Then use your choice of colored media, and use colors, abstract shapes, or symbols to indicate the specific factors or relevant feelings within each piece of pie. Try to refrain from writing words on the pie itself, and instead make a separate "legend" or table at the bottom of the page to describe your pie chart. Feel free to be creative and adjust this project to make it work for you! We'll share our results later in the session.

Handout for clients: Biopsychosocial-spiritual (BPSS) descriptions for pie chart activity

Biological aspects include the physical effects on your body. Can you sense whether you have a physiological dependence on your habit? Do you experience intense cravings or responses to cues or triggers? Have you noticed any kind of tolerance (you can handle more of the drug than you used to) or withdrawal symptoms? Consider things like the impact on your health, any automotive accidents caused by being high, other types of accidents and injuries, etc. You may also refer to etiology. Do you think there are genetic components to your issue?

Psychological aspects include mental or emotional reliance on your drug to relieve stress or medicate unpleasant feelings. You might use your drug to provide courage to face a task; or ease discomfort in a social, academic, work, or sexual situation; or comfort yourself after a stressful event. For some people, using might be about celebrating, whether it's a special event or the arrival of the weekend. Or you might have latched on to your drug just because it made you feel so good when you tried it.

In this slice, you could also include cognitive factors that you might have learned about in treatment, such as your personal locus of control (whether you tend to attribute success and failure to yourself or to outside factors—do you respond to failure by trying harder, or by blaming others, giving up, or getting high?) and self-talk (exaggerating the hassle of everyday negative events, personalizing events that are not about you, etc.—which you might identify as related to your drug use).

Social aspects refer to your relationships, lifestyle, family influences, social circle or subculture, academic or work environment, etc. For example, certain behaviors or habits may be expected in some settings, and you may have to explain or not be accepted if you do *not* want to participate. Sometimes a person has a minor habit that becomes more severe because a friend or partner wants them to drink or use at the same (higher) level. Other environmental factors might include living in a house where there is always partying going on, or working in a bar or other place where drug activity takes place. Broader cultural expectations might include an expectation that if you're a man, you should be able to drink heavily and hold your liquor, or if a woman, that you accept drinks offered by a man even if you feel you're at your limit for the night. When you think of etiology, you might think of the influence your parents' or other family members' alcohol and other drug (AOD) use had on you. The availability of your drug is another environmental factor you could address here if you wish.

Spiritual aspects refer to beliefs, values, and finding meaning in life—whether or not you consider yourself religious. Is your AOD use creating a contradiction between the morals or values you hold (or once held) and your current behaviors? Do you feel a kind of emptiness, such as wondering why you should bother to change anyway, or shame, such as a sense that you are just too bad a person to change? Did you use out of hopelessness or despair? Remember, the pie chart is to show which components go into creating or maintaining your addictive behavior. Sometimes people feel that a spiritual experience has helped them to *stop* using, so that wouldn't be included unless you were making a pie about your strengths for recovery.

The assertiveness continuum and storyboard (Chapter 5)

Group approaches are effective for building skills in being *assertive*, which can be conceptualized as being in the middle of a continuum, being neither *passive* (going along, even against one's better judgment) nor *aggressive* (responding in a way that offends others or infringes upon their rights). Passive-aggressive behavior is a form of aggressive behavior that may not overtly appear to be so, for example, agreeing to give someone a ride to work when you have no intention of following through, or giving a backhanded compliment.

For the basic storyboard activity, clients are given four sheets of paper. They first come up with a challenging situation where they would want to say no but have difficulty doing so, such as an old friend being in town for a visit and asking them out for a drink. This is shown in the first picture in the strip. Then, three alternative possible ways of responding are depicted on the remaining pages, to portray a passive, aggressive (or passive-aggressive), and assertive manner of responding. Most drug treatment programs teach refusal skills that can be reviewed and employed for the assertive response.

The directive can stop here, or clients can be given three additional pieces of paper and asked to depict the three likely outcomes of their three responses, including how they would feel about themselves. Group processing of the storyboards can give individuals ideas for new responses or feedback about probable outcomes. Facilitators can encourage impromptu role-play to solidify learning from the storyboard.

The mountaintop self-portrait (Chapter 5)

Group or individual art therapy activities that provide a sense of play or fun are important to include on occasion. This directive can be a tool for personalizing and recalling the sense of perspective gained by the mountain guided imagery described in Chapter 5. Verbal processing of this directive can focus on these and other topics, such as, "What sort of things motivate you to persevere when you have a 'steep road ahead'?" Have you ever accomplished something that took a really long time? The facilitator might also recommend an affirmation such as: *My vision has been limited by my addiction, but now I know there is much more to the world than I had ever imagined. The whole world will open up to me if I persist in my journey to the top.*

The most satisfying way to create this directive involves use of a photographic self-image. The art therapist would need to discuss with the agency administration whether and how clients can be photographed for this purpose. Having the clients draw themselves at the top of the mountain is an alternative, although this does not seem to be as engaging or effective. Use of photographic self-portraits is often a good fit for those with natural narcissism like adolescents and people with addiction issues (PWAI); however, some people in drug treatment may be reluctant if their drug use has resulted in negative changes in appearance. While it is important to be aware of this possibility, clients can be encouraged to view this as a way to reframe themselves in a fun way. An example of a mountaintop drawing is shown in Figure AA.1, with the head altered for the client's confidentiality.

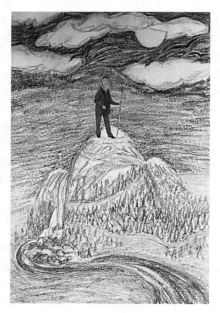

Figure AA.1: Mountaintop self-portrait (see color plate)

Explain to the group that this activity involves individually posing for a photo, which will then be sized and printed on paper, cut out, and glued onto a drawing, and the digital photograph deleted. Offer to step outside or into a hallway to take the picture if clients feel self-conscious posing in front of the group. In addition to a digital camera or phone, this directive requires a computer with a program to size the photos, and a color printer. Depending on the session length and other considerations, this directive may need to be done over two sessions, allowing time between sessions for the facilitator to prepare the photos, or clients can be assisted to do this. Before taking the photos, encourage clients to determine the metaphorical intention or goal for their mountain journey, or to imagine their feelings at the top of a mountain; you may wish to suggest possibilities such as awe, amazement, triumph, joy, accomplishment, and wonder. Clients are then photographed individually, with a facial and bodily expression of their choice to convey their feeling. When they are satisfied with the photo, it is downloaded and sized so that the person is in a caricature proportion to the top of a mountain landscape on the given page size. Images of clients in the same group should be sized similarly. The clients then cut out their figure from the background in the photo.

A vertically oriented paper with elongated dimensions (e.g., 12" × 18", rather than a more squarish rectangle) serves to emphasize the height of the mountains and the journey upward. It also seems to make planning the drawing less difficult for clients. After drawing the personal mountain scene, the figure is glued atop.

This has been a popular directive in my experience, with a higher-than-usual number of clients retaining their drawings to take home. These drawings can also be displayed together as a group mural that mirrors the group cohesion by depicting them as successful mountain climbers together.

Themes for paper wall quilts (Chapter 5)

Lists of topics for individual drawings that can be incorporated into themed paper quilts, as described in Chapter 5, follow. These are sample lists that can be adjusted to make a certain size quilt. Time should be given in group to brainstorm lists and identify personal spins on the individual topics. Symbolic, representational, or abstract depictions can be labeled or captioned to create the finished quilt block. Markers or oil pastels and 12" × 12" multimedia drawing paper are recommended. I encourage participants to design their blocks so that color is present throughout the square; in other words, even if they are starting with a line drawing, to color in all the elements, including the background. This creates the stronger design and more appealing look of an actual fabric quilt.

Quilt theme: Rationale for total abstinence

Many clients struggle with the thought that they have to give up all psychoactive drugs, even those that they do not perceive as problematic for them. This quilt is a good way of reinforcing these concepts.

1. Cross-addiction means you can quickly become just as dependent if you switch to another drug, particularly one in the same pharmacological category (e.g., benzodiazepines for alcohol).
2. Use of other drugs/alcohol can trigger use of drug of choice because of associative conditioning.
3. The act of using any drug triggers thinking about the drug of choice.
4. Willpower and judgment are greatly reduced when you are high on anything.
5. Using other drugs means you are probably still using drugs to:
   a. emotionally medicate
   b. avoid stress, conflict, or facing problems
   c. not grow or mature.
6. Staying with the same playmates or playgrounds leads to relapse to drug of choice.
7. Diminished identification with personal values or spirituality.
8. No sense of accomplishment of building sobriety over time.
9. Continuation of guilt- and shame-based behaviors and effects on others.

Quilt theme: Relapse triggers or barriers to recovery

1. Euphoric recall (thinking only about the best times you were high).
2. Becoming emotionally involved in a new relationship too soon (even a seemingly good one).
3. Enabling another or directing most or all of your attention to someone else.
4. Loneliness, isolation, or withdrawal from those who would help.

5. Uncontrolled feelings.

6. Over-controlled (repressed) feelings.

7. Over-involvement: becoming obsessed with filling up your time.

8. Forgetting the disease process and thinking you could use just a little now and then.

9. Indulging in self-pity: poor me, why me?

10. Not keeping things in perspective; overreacting.

11. Rationalizing unhealthy behaviors.

12. Impatience; need for instant gratification.

13. Boredom.

14. Focusing on others' problems.

15. Dishonesty.

16. High-stress lifestyle.

17. Using nonassertive (passive or aggressive) means to express feelings and get needs met.

18. Procrastination on needed tasks.

19. Wanting to celebrate; thinking you deserve to use.

20. Unresolved grief or past abuse.

Mapping internal and external triggers *and* creating a trigger-safe environment (Chapter 6)

Art therapist Leslie Woodruff articulated this directive idea in a lesson plan format to meet needs at her workplace, a substance abuse unit in an acute care behavioral health hospital (Woodruff, personal communication 2016). Part of the generic treatment plan at the unit was for clients to examine personal triggers for problematic substance use. Woodruff noted that her body-map trigger drawing was an effective learning tool; however, this crisis population often found that making the drawings was itself triggering. To provide safety and avoid leaving clients feeling vulnerable at the end of the group, she added a second directive—a special version of a safe place drawing that uses the same foldover doors format as the secret garden (see Chapter 7). She noted that this lesson plan was used only in sessions of sufficient length to allow both pieces to be completed. Art therapists may find it helpful when advocating for group time by showing employers directives that are described in this kind of format, with identified objectives and discussion points. This outline also provides bulleted lecture points about types of triggers, which are likely to prompt personal examples from participants.

Objective: Clients learn to identify internal and external triggers to help prevent relapse, and to conceptualize a safe or trigger-free environment.

Time: Group session of 90 minutes or more.

Materials: Predrawn generic body outline on copy paper, blank white copy paper, 12" × 18" construction paper in various colors, markers or oil pastels, glue.

Procedure:

0–10 minutes: Art therapist leads a discussion about internal and external triggers. Clients brainstorm personal examples with each other. Here are a few:

- *Internal triggers:* anxiety; excitement; boredom; frustration; grief; insecurity; physical pain; good or bad memories; trauma or drug-related flashbacks.

- *External triggers:* Being around certain friends; hearing certain music; going on a trip or vacation; being home alone; attending business functions or celebrations; driving by a bar or liquor store; being in a car; seeing a movie where drug use is portrayed.

10–30 minutes: Using the body outline prompt and markers or oil pastels, clients depict external triggers in the space outside the body outline, and internal triggers inside the body outline.

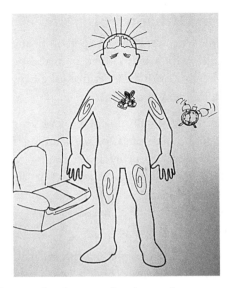

Figure AA.2: In this exemplar, the person drew her couch as an external location trigger; the alarm clock is an unpleasant reminder of daily responsibilities; boxing gloves to the heart represent upset feelings; external strike marks toward the brain represent stressors and mental agitation; spirals on arms and legs represent feeling sluggish; and bags under the eyes symbolize not being able to sleep

30–45 minutes: Clients share their triggers and generate ideas for avoiding, combating, or distracting themselves from them.

45–75 minutes: Clients then use the blank white paper oriented in the portrait position to draw a fantasy environment that would be free from triggers or that would actively address triggers effectively. When done, they choose a color of construction paper, and with it placed in the landscape position, fold in both ends toward the center line to create a double door that will cover the trigger-free environment drawing. The doors are embellished as desired; they may be fanciful and inviting, or heavily guarded. The drawing of the trigger-free place is glued on the inside where it is kept safe.

75–90 minutes: Discuss this experience. Suggest that clients practice envisioning their trigger-free place whenever they feel triggered. At home, they may want to keep their drawings somewhere where they will view them regularly. Ask whether the trigger drawing is itself triggering. If so, what is a good response to it? (Perhaps to glue it to the back of the folded construction paper of the safe place assembly.)

Your inner critic (Chapter 6)

This is a directive that requires clients to personify and externalize their disparaging self-talk, which helps them gain the perspective needed to observe and challenge or disconnect from their own negativity. The facilitator may use this text as a script.

> People in early recovery usually do not think very highly of themselves. You may be feeling guilt, shame, or self-loathing. Sometimes people become their own worst enemy by repeating thoughts like: "No matter what I do, I always mess things up," or "I'll never be able to stay sober, I'm such a loser," or "I don't deserve to have a good life." When you mentally repeat these messages, they erode your sense of hope and your ability to change.
>
> A technique that is helpful in quieting this self-talk is to think of the destructive internal messages as coming from a part of yourself called the inner critic. This is not the same as your conscience or healthy guilt. Your inner critic may replay shaming tapes you've heard from other people at different times in your life, or just have a life of its own related to your addiction.
>
> Once you recognize the destructive power of your inner critic as something apart from the rest of you, it is easier to challenge it. You do not need to have your inner critic continue to tell you that you are an unworthy human being. When it talks, you can learn to picture it, then challenge or ignore it. Work on proving it wrong, and soon it will begin to fade away.
>
> For this activity, start by identifying your inner critic's most common messages. Jot them down on a piece of paper. Next, draw a picture or use collage images to create your inner critic. Be creative…maybe you will combine facial or body parts from different magazine images, or draw your inner critic as a certain kind of animal. If you're not sure how to start, close your eyes, and imagine the voice saying something. Now start drawing or looking for the right images. When you're satisfied that you have made a convincing picture, think of how you can talk back to this critic and challenge the messages you wrote down. Write out your responses. Later today or tomorrow, whenever that voice pops into your head again, picture where it's coming from and challenge the message. You can also ignore it, or you can practice saying, "Oh, it's just you again!" and go about the rest of your day.

Replication, Re-vision, and Reflection (RRR) (Chapter 8)

This is not a client directive, but a technique for the art therapist's use. By replicating client artwork, art therapists can bypass or explore countertransference reactions or stereotyped interpretations.

Foundation: the client and the client's drawing

This technique is not particularly helpful for use with children or with those with cognitive impairments, whether these are due to disabilities, organicity, or psychosis. It is best to use a directed drawing that does not have an overt emotional challenge, such as a bridge drawing or Kinetic House-Tree-Person (K-H-T-P) drawing. You need to have observed the drawing as it was being created, because you will try to replicate the client's drawing sequence and style (speed, level of concentration, affective display, body language, etc.).

Performing the RRR

Do the RRR when you are alone:

1. *Replication:* By looking at the original drawing, copy it as accurately as possible. Try to draw the elements in the same order and in the same attitude that the client did. Do not refer to session notes or perform another simultaneous activity. Keep your mental activity to a minimum: *notice, but do not stop to judge or analyze*, any thoughts or feelings that bubble up as you draw, as if you were the client making the drawing.

2. *Re-vision:* Make a new drawing by drawing the same general picture, but changing or strengthening fragile or discordant aspects. You may add or delete minor elements. Again, let the activity flow, minimizing in-depth analysis and allowing for serendipity.

3. *Reflection:* Reflect in writing on this process. Address the thoughts and feelings noted as you replicated the drawing and as you created the re-vision. As you bring in the more verbal and analytical processing, you may identify further insights into the client.

Caveats

Even though this may have been an authentic-seeming experience, never take action (such as changing a treatment plan) that could adversely affect your client, should your interpretation be wrong. Also, I do not recommend that you process this with the client unless you first carefully consider the range of possible outcomes and discuss the idea with a supervisor or knowledgeable colleague. Negative consequences include being erroneous in your interpretation, or the client's displeasure at the thought of you doing this process without their knowledge. Conversely, if the therapeutic relationship has been established, it might be seen as a sign of caring that you took the time to do this to try to better understand the client.

The family forest task (Chapter 9)

Research and theory in both family therapy and addictions has tended to focus on the prototypical definition of an intact nuclear family with an identifiable bloodline. However, clinical use of this definition has been criticized for its narrow alignment with the white Anglo-Saxon Protestant cultural ideal (Stevens and Smith 2013). In SAT, it is not unusual to see clients who do not know their fathers, were raised by people other than their biological parents, or who have experienced incest or other traumatic family issues. Those in such families can feel confused, ashamed, or distressed when given art therapy tasks based on traditional family trees or genograms. Johnson (2004) recommended a phenomenological approach for substance abuse counselors wherein "family" is defined as the people whom clients consider to be members of their family, regardless of legal, blood, or geographical ties.

Arrington, author of *Home Is Where the Art Is* (2001), titled a brief subsection in her book's appendix "The National Forest" (p.206). In discussing the value of creating genograms or family trees in family art therapy, she noted that many families have tangled interconnections due to divorces, remarriages, adoptions, foster placements, and similar situations. Arrington suggested viewing family relationships as a forest, with a variety of specimens that share the same environment. She wrote, "Within the general symbol of landscape, forests occupy a notable place, and are often found in myths, legends, and folktales. A forest is a dense growth of trees and underbrush connected on all levels with the Great Mother" (2001, p. 206).

Although she made a useful and inspiring point, Arrington did not create a specific directive or expound on the meaning of her term *national forest*. The word *national* does convey expansiveness and the idea of extended family; however, for some, it may suggest a political and possibly paternalistic attribute that does not particularly align with archetypal associations to the forest and the Great Mother. This feminine archetypal imagery is comforting because it sends a subconscious message that differences are just fine; they are part of the natural order. Unlike a linear patriarchal system that is defined by pedigrees and disavows nonlegalized relationships, Mother Nature is *not* perfectly orderly. A forest does have "tangled undergrowth" that is an accepted, natural, and vital part of its identity.

Inspired by Arrington's notion, I implemented a family forest task. One of the goals is to help a family create an aesthetically pleasing "group portrait," and to that end I restrict choice of media to oil pastels or crayons, which allow blending, shading, and strength of color. Most clients do not achieve the same depth of pigment when they use colored pencils, and in general, I have found that markers tend to result in more rapid, cartoonish depictions and less in-depth involvement with a task.

Pre-adolescents and some older clients may not possess the abstract cognitive ability or imagination to symbolize their personal characteristics in a tree. As part of an informal family assessment process using this directive, it is important to observe whether and how older family members attempt to interpret the task to help the younger client. If no such help is forthcoming and the child appears confused, the therapist can suggest alternative directions such as *if you could be any tree you wanted, what tree would you be? What would your tree look like?* or simply, *draw your favorite kind of tree*. The words "any you wanted" or "favorite" ensure that the product will reflect a positive focus, to parallel the strengths focus of the standard direction. When family members have finished creating their trees, they are asked to set them aside momentarily. They are then asked to work together to make trees to depict other people they wish to include in the family, each a tree on its own piece of paper. The concluding activity is to have the family decide how to place all the tree images in relationship to each other (on mural paper, the floor, or tacked to a wall), thus creating the family forest, and to reflect together on this process. The therapist should make a photographic record of the final arrangement. The value of this task can be renewed later in therapy, when symbolic changes in position are made to reflect the evolving family relationships. Family members may even want to modify or redraw their trees or those of others, to indicate growth or strengths gained.

Variation for groups

Art therapist Alison Boughn (personal communication June 2015) developed a forest directive for use in SAT groups. Each person identified their own personal strengths and characteristics by talking with the others. Each then drew a tree representing those strengths, and placed it as desired to create a group forest. This directive has value for the clients in the therapeutic experience, and Boughn reported that it was accessible and popular. In addition, the products and observation of group dynamics contain informal assessment value for the art therapist.

Appendix B
Resources About Substance Abuse

Useful organizations

The following reliable nonprofit and governmental agency websites provide a wealth of information about substance abuse treatment (SAT) best practices, drugs of abuse, news regarding scientific and legislative issues, and related issues. These sources provide news services, newsletters, books, white papers, educational materials, webinars, research support, and more, many of them free or nominally priced. (See the List of Acronyms in the Introduction if needed.)

CSAT/SAMHSA—a variety of excellent publications

http://store.samhsa.gov/home

NAADAC—webinars, continuing-education publications

www.naadac.org

NCADD—newsletter, referrals, advocacy

www.ncadd.org

NIDA—educational materials, research grants

www.drugabuse.gov

Partnership for Drug-Free Kids—news service; not limited to children's issues

http://drugfree.org/learn/drug-and-alcohol-news

Quick and easy desk references

Streetdrugs.org (2016) *Streetdrugs: A Drug Identification Guide*. Berkeley, CA: Publisher's Group West. Available directly from www.streetdrugs.org

This inexpensive handbook produced by a nonprofit features color photos on each page with descriptions of drugs of abuse, including the most recent versions or designer drugs. It is updated annually using information and photographs from drug interdiction and treatment sources, and is used by law enforcement and other professionals.

Kuhn, C., Swartzwelder, S., and Wilson, W. (2014) *Buzzed: The Straight Facts About the Most Used and Abused Drugs from Alcohol to Ecstasy*. New York: W.W. Norton. (Original work published 1998.)

Mooney, A.J., Dold, C., and Eisenberg, H. (2014) *The Recovery Book: Answers to All Your Questions About Addiction and Alcoholism and Finding Health and Happiness in Sobriety*. New York: Workman. (Original work published 1992.)

These two books are highly recommended as convenient references for anyone, from those in recovery to their partners or families, students, and professionals. They are relatively inexpensive, well organized, and easy to read, yet authoritative. Both are updated regularly, so look for the most recent editions.

C., R. (2012) *The Little Book: A Collection of Alternative 12 Steps*. Toronto: AA Agnostica.

A fascinating and helpful look at variations on the Twelve Steps that address the particular needs of women, Native Americans, Buddhists, atheists, and others.

Specialty publishers

Hazelden Publishing—probably the oldest and best-known independent publisher of materials about addiction and recovery, including workbooks and manuals, which are widely used by providers and recovering people alike.

> www.hazelden.org/web/public/store.page

The AA and NA World Services offices provide a range of their own literature.

> Alcoholics Anonymous World Services
>
> www.aa.org/pages/en_US/aa-literature

Narcotics Anonymous World Services

www.na.org/?ID=literature

Professional journals

This is not an exhaustive list; consult a university library for further assistance.

Addiction Research & Theory

www.tandfonline.com/loi/iart20

Alcohol Research & Health

https://pubs.niaaa.nih.gov/publications/arh341/toc34_1.htm

Journal of Addictive Diseases

www.tandfonline.com/loi/wjad20

Journal of Ethnicity in Substance Abuse

www.tandfonline.com/loi/wesa20

Journal of Psychoactive Drugs

www.tandfonline.com/loi/ujpd20

Journal of Social Work Practice in the Addictions

www.tandfonline.com/loi/wswp20

Journal of Substance Abuse and Alcoholism

www.jscimedcentral.com/SubstanceAbuse

Journal of Substance Abuse Treatment

www.journals.elsevier.com/journal-of-substance-abuse-treatment

Substance Abuse

www.tandfonline.com/loi/wsub20

Substance Abuse: Research and Treatment

http://insights.sagepub.com/substance-abuse-research-and-treatment-journal-j80

Self-help groups

In addition to these national websites, local AA and NA sites are readily found with Google searches, and provide information about meeting times and locations.

Alcoholics Anonymous®

www.aa.org

Narcotics Anonymous®

www.na.org

Recommended nonspiritual self-help organizations include:

SOS (Secular Organizations for Sobriety)

www.sossobriety.org

SMART Recovery® (Self Management And Recovery Training)

www.smartrecovery.org

References

AA (Alcoholics Anonymous) (2001) *Alcoholics Anonymous*. New York: Alcoholics Anonymous World Services (original work published 1939).

AA (2010) *Alcoholics Anonymous Comes of Age*. New York: Alcoholics Anonymous World Services (original work published 1957).

Adedoyin, C., Burns, N., Jackson, H.M., and Franklin, S. (2014) 'Revisiting holistic interventions in substance abuse treatment.' *Journal of Human Behavior in the Social Environment 24*, 538–546.

Adelman, E. and Castricone, L. (1986) 'An expressive arts model for substance abuse group training and treatment.' *The Arts in Psychotherapy 13*, 1, 53–59.

Albert-Puleo, N. (1980) 'Modern psychoanalytic art therapy and its application to drug abuse.' *The Arts in Psychotherapy 7*, 1, 43–52.

Albert-Puleo, N. and Osha, V. (1976–77, Winter) 'Art therapy as an alcoholism treatment tool.' *Alcohol Health and Research World*, 28–31.

Alberts, A., Elkind, D., and Ginsberg, S. (2007) 'The personal fable and risk-taking in early adolescence.' *Journal of Youth and Adolescence 36*, 1.

Aletraris, L., Paino, M., Edmond, M.B., Roman, P.M., and Bride, B.E. (2014) 'The use of art and music therapy in substance abuse treatment programs.' *Journal of Addictions Nursing 25*, 4, 190–196.

Allen, P. (1985) 'Integrating art therapy into an alcoholism treatment program.' *American Journal of Art Therapy 24*, 1, 10–12.

Angheluta, A.M. and Lee, B.K. (2011) 'Art therapy for chronic pain: Applications and future directions.' *Canadian Journal of Counselling and Psychotherapy 45*, 2, 112–131.

APA (American Psychiatric Association) (2013) *Diagnostic and Statistical Manual of Mental Disorders, 5th Edition*. Arlington, VA: APA.

Arrington, D.B. (2001) *Home Is Where the Art Is: An Art Therapy Approach to Family Therapy*. Springfield, IL: Charles C. Thomas.

ASAM (American Society of Addiction Medicine) (2011) *Public Policy Statement: Definition of Addiction*. Available at www.asam.org/quality-practice/definition-of-addiction, accessed on January 23, 2016.

ASAM (2016) *The ASAM Criteria*. Available at www.asam.org/quality-practice/guidelines-and-consensus-documents/the-asam-criteria/about, accessed on September 13, 2016.

ATCB (Art Therapy Credentials Board, Inc.) (2016 rev.) *ATCB Code of Ethics, Conduct, and Disciplinary Procedures.* Available at www.atcb.org/Ethics/ATCBCode, accessed on January 12, 2016.

Ault, R.E. (ca. 1976) 'Paper on Drugs–Hippy Culture.' Unpublished manuscript, Emporia, KS: Department of Counselor Education, Emporia State University.

Barry, D. and Petry, N.M. (2009) 'Cognitive Behavioral Treatments for Substance Use Disorders.' In P.M. Miller (ed.) *Evidence-Based Addiction Treatment* (pp.159–174). New York: Academic Press.

Bellwood, L.R. (1975, Spring) 'Grief work in alcoholism treatment.' *Alcohol Health and Research World* 8–11.

Biley, F.C. (2006) 'The arts, literature, and the attraction paradigm: Changing attitudes toward substance misuse service users.' *Journal of Substance Use 11,* 1, 11–21.

Black, C. (1981) *It Will Never Happen to Me.* Denver, CO: MAC.

Blos, P. (1962) *On Adolescence.* New York: Free Press.

Booth, L. (1991) *When God Becomes a Drug.* New York: Tarcher.

Bowen, S., Chawla, N., and Marlatt, A. (2011) *Mindfulness-based Relapse Prevention for Addictive Behaviors.* New York: Guilford Press.

Bowlby, J. (1988) *A Secure Base: Parent–Child Attachment and Healthy Human Development.* New York: Basic Books.

Breslin, K.T., Reed, M.R., and Malone, S.B. (2003) 'An holistic approach to substance abuse treatment.' *Journal of Psychoactive Drugs 35,* 2, 247–251.

Bricker, M. (2014) *A Primer on Attachment, Trauma, and Substance Use Disorders.* NAADAC webinar. Available at www.naadac.org/webinars, accessed on October 23, 2014.

Brooke, S.L. (ed) (2009) *The Use of Creative Therapies with Chemical Dependency Issues.* Springfield, IL: Charles C. Thomas.

Burns, R.C. (1987) *Kinetic-House-Tree-Person Drawings (K-H-T-P): An Interpretative Manual.* New York: Brunner/Mazel.

Burns, R.C. and Kaufman, S.H. (1972) *Actions, Styles and Symbols in Kinetic Family Drawings (K-F-D).* New York: Brunner/Mazel.

C., R. (2012) *The Little Book: A Collection of Alternative 12 Steps.* Toronto, ON: AA Agnostica.

Callaghan, G.M. (1993) 'Art Therapy with Alcoholic Families.' In D. Linesch (ed.) *Art Therapy with Families in Crisis* (pp.69–103). New York: Brunner/Mazel.

Cameron, J. (2002) *The Artist's Way: A Spiritual Path to Higher Creativity.* New York: Tarcher (original work published 1992).

Canty, J. (2009) 'The key to being in the right mind.' *International Journal of Art Therapy 14,* 1, 11–16.

Capuzzi, D. and Stauffer, M.D. (2016) *Foundations of Addictions Counseling.* Boston, MA: Pearson (original work published 2008).

Carolan, R. (2007) 'Adolescents, Identity, Addiction, and Imagery.' In D.B. Arrington (ed.) *Art, Angst, and Trauma: Right Brain Interventions with Developmental Issues* (pp.99–115). Springfield, IL: Charles C. Thomas.

CDC (Centers for Disease Control and Prevention) (2014) *Opioid Painkiller Prescribing*. Atlanta, GA: CDC. Available at www.cdc.gov/vitalsigns/opioid-prescribing, accessed on August 6, 2016.

Chamberlain, L.L. (2013) 'Assessment and Diagnosis.' In P. Stevens and R.L. Smith (eds) *Substance Abuse Counseling: Theory and Practice* (5th edn) (pp.122–154). Upper Saddle River, NJ: Pearson Education.

Chickerneo, N.B. (1993) *Portraits of Spirituality in Recovery: The Use of Art in Recovery from Codependency and/or Chemical Dependency*. Springfield, IL: Charles C. Thomas.

Chilton, G. and Wilkinson, R. (2015) *Low-Key Joy*. Available at http://creativewellbeingworkshops.com/2015/04/low-key-joy, accessed on December 28, 2015.

Cicero, T.J., Ellis, M.S., Surratt, H.L., and Kurtz, S.P. (2014) 'The changing face of heroin use in the United States.' *JAMA Psychiatry 71*, 7, 821–826.

Colgate, V. (2016) 'Shadows of Resistance: An Art Directive for Substance Abuse Treatment.' Unpublished Master's project. Emporia, KS: Emporia State University.

Conger, D. (1988) 'Suicidal youth: The challenge to art therapy.' *American Journal of Art Therapy 27*, 34–44.

Connors, G.J., DiClemente, C.C., Velasquez, M.M., and Donovan, D.M. (2013) *Substance Abuse Treatment and the Stages of Change*. New York: Guilford Press.

Cox, K.L. and Price, K. (1990) 'Breaking through: Incident drawings with adolescent substance abusers.' *The Arts in Psychotherapy 17*, 333–337.

Crowe, A. and Parmenter, A.S. (2012) 'Creative approaches to motivational interviewing: Addressing the principles.' *Journal of Creativity in Mental Health 7*, 124–140.

CSAT (Center for Substance Abuse Treatment) (1999) *Treatment Improvement Protocol (TIP) Series, 35: Enhancing Motivation for Change in Substance Abuse Treatment*. Rockville, MD: SAMHSA (Substance Abuse and Mental Health Services Administration). Available at https://store.samhsa.gov/shin/content/SMA13-4212/SMA13-4212.pdf, accessed on March 8, 2017.

CSAT (2005) *TIP Series, 41: Substance Abuse Treatment: Group Therapy*. Rockville, MD: SAMHSA (Substance Abuse and Mental Health Services Administration).

Csikszentmihalyi, M. (1991) *Flow: The Psychology of Optimal Experience*. New York: Harper Perennial.

Devine, D. (1970) 'A preliminary investigation of paintings by alcoholic men.' *American Journal of Art Therapy 9*, 3, 115–128.

Dickman, S.B., Dunn, J.E., and Wolf, A. (1996) 'The use of art therapy as a predictor of relapse in chemical dependency treatment.' *Art Therapy 13*, 4, 232–237.

Dickson, C. (2007) 'An evaluation study of art therapy provision in a residential Addiction Treatment Programme (ATP).' *International Journal of Art Therapy 12*, 1, 17–27.

Diehls, V.A. (2008) 'Art Therapy, Substance Abuse, and the Stages of Change.' Unpublished Master's thesis. Emporia, KS: Emporia State University.

Donnenberg, D. (1978) 'Art therapy in a drug community.' *Confinia Psychiatrica* 21, 37–44.

Dore, E.A. (2012) 'Posttraumatic stress disorder, depression and suicidality in inpatients with substance abuse disorders.' *Drug and Alcohol Review 31*, 3, 294–302.

DuWors, G. (2013) 'The mindful practices of Alcoholics Anonymous.' *Advances in Addiction and Recovery 1*, 4, 28–30.

Ellis, A. and Dryden, W. (2007) *The Practice of Rational Emotive Behavior Therapy.* New York: Springer (original work published 1997).

Emunah, R. (1990) 'Expression and expansion in adolescence: The significance of creative arts therapy.' *The Arts in Psychotherapy 17*, 101–107.

Engel, G.L. (1977) 'The need for a new medical model: A challenge for biomedicine.' *Science 196*, 129–136.

Erdmann, G.W. (1972) 'Painting Helps Alcoholic Bring His Problems into Focus' (case vignette). In J.C. Coleman (ed.) *Abnormal Psychology and Modern Life* (pp.182–183). Glenview, IL: Scott, Foresman.

Erikson, E. (1994) *Identity and the Life Cycle.* New York: W.W. Norton (original work published 1959).

Faulkner, C.A. (2013) 'Etiology of Substance Abuse: Why People Use.' In P.W. Stevens and R.L. Smith (eds) *Substance Abuse Counseling: Theory and Practice* (5th edn) (pp.98–121). Upper Saddle River, NJ: Pearson Education.

Feen-Calligan, H. (1995) 'The use of art therapy in treatment programs to promote spiritual recovery from addiction.' *Art Therapy 12*, 1, 46–50.

Feen-Calligan, H. (1999) 'Enlightenment in Chemical Dependency Treatment Programs: A Grounded Theory.' In C.A. Malchiodi (ed.) *Medical Art Therapy with Adults* (pp.137–162). London: Jessica Kingsley Publishers.

Feen-Calligan, H. (2007) 'The use of art therapy in detoxification from chemical addiction.' *Canadian Art Therapy Association Journal 20*, 1, 16–28.

Feen-Calligan, H., Washington, O.G.M., and Moxley, D.P. (2008) 'Use of artwork as a visual processing modality in group treatment of chemically dependent minority women.' *The Arts in Psychotherapy 35*, 4, 287–295.

Felitti, V.J., Anda, R.F., Nordenberg, D., Williamson, D.F. *et al.* (1998) 'Relationship of childhood abuse and household dysfunction to many of the leading causes of death in adults: The Adverse Childhood Experiences (ACE) study.' *American Journal of Preventative Medicine 14*, 4, 245–258.

Fernandez, K.M. (2009) 'Comic Addict: A Qualitative Study of the Benefits of Addressing Ambivalence through Comic/Cartoon Drawing with Clients in In-patient Treatment for Chemical Dependency.' In S.L. Brooke (ed.) *The Use of Creative Therapies with Chemical Dependency Issues* (pp.80–105). Springfield, IL: Charles C. Thomas.

Flores, P.J. (2004) *Addiction as an Attachment Disorder.* Lanham, MD: James Aronson.

Forrest, G. (1975) 'The problems of dependency and the value of art therapy as a means of treating alcoholism.' *Art Psychotherapy 2*, 1, 15–43.

Fosha, D., Siegel, D.J., and Solomon, M.F. (eds) (2009) *The Healing Power of Emotions: Affective Neuroscience, Development, and Clinical Practice.* New York: Norton.

Foulke, W. and Keller, T. (1976) 'The art experience in addict rehabilitation.' *American Journal of Art Therapy 15*, 3, 75–80.

Francis, D., Kaiser, D., and Deaver, S. (2003) 'Representations of attachment security in the Bird's Nest Drawings of clients with substance abuse disorders.' *Art Therapy 20*, 3, 125–137.

Fredrickson, B.L. (2009) *Positivity.* New York: Crown.

Furth, G.M. (2002) *The Secret World of Drawings.* Toronto, ON: Inner City Books.

Gantt, L.M. (2001) 'The Formal Elements Art Therapy Scale: A measurement system for global variables in art.' *Art Therapy 18*, 1, 50–55.

Gantt, L. and Tabone, C. (1998) *The Formal Elements Art Therapy Scale: Rating Manual.* Morgantown, WV: Gargoyle Press.

Gerber, N. (2016) 'Mixed Methods Research and Art Therapy.' In D.E. Gussak and M.L. Rosal (eds) *The Wiley Handbook of Art Therapy* (pp.654–663). Chichester: John Wiley & Sons.

Gerity, L.A. (2001) 'Josie, Winnicott, and the hungry ghosts.' *Art Therapy 18*, 1, 44–49.

Glidden, K. and Brown, J. (2016, June) 'Childhood Trauma and Addiction.' Paper presented at the NAADAC Behavioral Health Conference, Lincoln, NE.

Glover, N.M. (1999) 'Play therapy and art therapy for substance abuse clients who have a history of incest victimization.' *Journal of Substance Abuse Treatment 16*, 4, 281–287.

Golomb, C. (2004) *The Child's Creation of a Pictorial World.* Mahwah, NJ: Lawrence Erlbaum (original work published 1992).

Grof, C. (1993) *The Thirst for Wholeness: Attachment, Addiction, and the Spiritual Path.* New York: HarperCollins.

Groterath, A. (1999) 'Conceptions of Addiction and Implications for Treatment Approaches.' In D. Waller and J. Mahony (eds) *Treatment of Addiction: Current Issues for Arts Therapies* (pp.14–22). London: Routledge.

Groth-Marnat, G. and Wright, A.J. (2016) *Handbook of Psychological Assessment.* Hoboken, NJ: Wiley (original work published 1984).

Gutman, S.A. and Schindler, V.P. (2007) 'The neurological basis of occupation.' *Occupational Therapy International 14*, 2, 71–85.

Hagens, C.A. (2011) 'A Qualitative Study to Determine How Art Therapy May Benefit Women with Addictions Who Have Relapsed.' Master's thesis. Tallahassee, FL: Florida State University.

Haluzan, M. (2012) 'Art therapy in the treatment of alcoholics.' *Alcoholism: Journal on Alcoholism and Related Addictions 48*, 2, 99–105.

Hammer, E.F. (1958) *The Clinical Application of Projective Drawings.* Springfield, IL: Charles C. Thomas.

Hanes, M. (1995) 'Utilizing road drawings as a therapeutic metaphor in art therapy.' *American Journal of Art Therapy 34*, 1, 19–23.

Hanes, M.J. (2007) '"Face-to-face" with addiction: The spontaneous production of self-portraits in art therapy.' *Art Therapy 24*, 1, 33–36.

Hanson, R. (2013) *Hardwiring Happiness.* New York: Harmony Books.

Harms, E. (1973) 'Art therapy for the drug addict.' *Arts in Psychotherapy 1*, 55–59.

Hass-Cohen, N. and Carr, R. (eds) (2008) *Art Therapy and Clinical Neuroscience.* London: Jessica Kingsley Publishers.

Hayes, P.M. (2012) *Blending Art Therapy with the Twelve Steps of Alcoholics Anonymous: The Workbook.* Reseda, CA: Pamela M. Hayes.

Hays, P.A. (2016) *Addressing Cultural Complexities in Practice.* Washington, DC: American Psychological Association (original work published 1996).

Hays, R.E. and Lyons, S. (1981) 'The Bridge Drawing: A projective technique for assessment in art therapy.' *The Arts in Psychotherapy 8*, 207–217.

Head, V.B. (1975) 'Experiences with art therapy in short-term groups of day clinic addicted patients.' *The Ontario Psychologist 7*, 4, 42–49.

Heilig, M. (2015) *The Thirteenth Step: Addiction in the Age of Brain Science.* New York: Columbia University Press.

Hinz, L.D. (2009a) 'Order Out of Chaos: The Expressive Therapies Continuum as a Framework for Art Therapy Interventions in Substance Abuse Treatment.' In S.L. Brooke (ed.) *The Use of Creative Therapies with Chemical Dependency Issues* (pp.51–68). Springfield, IL: Charles C. Thomas.

Hinz, L.D. (2009b) *Expressive Therapies Continuum: A Framework for Using Art in Therapy.* New York: Routledge.

Holt, E. and Kaiser, D.H. (2001) 'Indicators of familial alcoholism in children's Kinetic Family Drawings.' *Art Therapy 18*, 2, 89–95.

Holt, E. and Kaiser, D.H. (2009) 'The First Step Series: Art therapy for early substance abuse treatment.' *The Arts in Psychotherapy 36*, 4, 245–250.

Horay, B.J. (2006) 'Moving towards gray: Art therapy and ambivalence in substance abuse treatment.' *Art Therapy 23*, 1, 14–22.

Horovitz, E.G. (2009) 'Combating Shame and Pathogenic Belief Systems: Theoretical and Art Therapy Applications for Chemical/Substance Abusive Deaf Clients.' In S.L. Brooke (ed.) *The Use of Creative Therapies with Chemical Dependency Issues* (pp.11–36). Springfield, IL: Charles C. Thomas.

Hoshino, J. (2008) 'Structural Family Art Therapy.' In C. Kerr, J. Hoshino, J. Sutherland, S.T. Parashak, and L.L. McCarley (eds) *Family Art Therapy: Foundations of Theory and Practice* (pp.119–150). New York: Routledge.

Hrenko, K.D. and Willis, R. (1996) 'The amusement park technique in the treatment of dually diagnosed psychiatric inpatients.' *Art Therapy 13*, 4, 261–264.

Hull, A. (2002) 'Neuroimaging findings in post-traumatic stress disorder: Systematic review.' *British Journal of Psychiatry 181*, 102–110.

Inaba, D.S. (2015) 'A scientific perspective on marijuana on the eve of its legalization.' *Advances in Addiction and Recovery 3*, 2, 21–25.

Johnson, D.R. (1990) 'Introduction to the special issue on creative arts therapies in the treatment of substance abuse.' *The Arts in Psychotherapy 17*, 295–298.

Johnson, J.L. (2004) *Fundamentals of Substance Abuse Practice.* Belmont, CA: Brooks/Cole.

Johnson, L. (1990) 'Creative therapies in the treatment of addictions: The art of transforming shame.' *The Arts in Psychotherapy 17,* 299–308.

Johnson, M.M. (2016) 'Cultural humility and sensitivity.' *Advances in Addiction and Recovery 26,* 3, 6–8.

Johnson, V. (1986) *Intervention: How to Help Someone Who Doesn't Want Help.* Center City, MN: Hazelden.

Jones, C.M. (2013) 'Heroin use and heroin use risk behaviors among nonmedical users of prescription opioid pain relievers.' *Drug and Alcohol Dependence 132,* 1, 95–100.

Julliard, K.N. (1995) 'Increasing chemically dependent patients' belief in Step One through expressive therapy.' *American Journal of Art Therapy 33,* 4, 110–119.

Julliard, K. (1999) *The Twelve Steps and Art Therapy* (monograph). Alexandria, VA: American Art Therapy Association.

Jung, C.G. (1963, January) 'Dr. C.G. Jung's reply to Bill W.'s letter.' *The Grapevine.* New York: Alcoholics Anonymous World Services (publication of personal letter written 1961).

Kagin, S.L. and Lusebrink, V.B. (1978) 'The Expressive Therapies Continuum.' *Art Psychotherapy 5,* 4, 171–180.

Kaiser, D. (1996) 'Indicators of attachment security in a drawing task.' *The Arts in Psychotherapy 23,* 4, 333–340.

Kaiser, D.H. and Deaver, S. (2009) 'Assessing attachment with the Bird's Nest Drawing: A review of the research.' *Art Therapy 26,* 1, 26–33.

Kasl, C.D. (1989) *Women, Sex, and Addiction.* New York: Harper & Row.

Kaufman, G.H. (1981) 'Art therapy with the addicted.' *Journal of Psychoactive Drugs 13,* 4, 353–360.

Khoury, L., Tang, Y.L., Bradley, B., Cubells, J.F., and Ressler, K.J. (2010) 'Substance use, childhood traumatic experience, and posttraumatic stress disorder.' *Depression and Anxiety 27,* 1077–1086.

Korb, A. (2012) 'The Grateful Brain.' *Psychology Today.* Available at www.psychologytoday.com/blog/prefrontal-nudity/201211/the-grateful-brain, accessed on November 15, 2016.

Krebs, K.A. (2008) 'Art Therapy Used to Enhance Steps One, Two, and Three of a Twelve-Step Recovery Program for Addictions Treatment.' Master's thesis. Pepper Pike, OH: Ursuline College.

Kuhn, C., Swartzwelder, S., and Wilson, W. (2014) *Buzzed: The Straight Facts About the Most Used and Abused Drugs from Alcohol to Ecstasy.* New York: W.W. Norton (original work published 1998).

Kurtz, E. (2008) *The Collected Ernie Kurtz.* New York: Author's Choice Press.

Kurtz, E. and Ketcham, K. (1992) *The Spirituality of Imperfection.* New York: Random House.

Lachman-Chapin, M. (1979) 'Kohut's theories on narcissism: Implications for art therapy.' *American Journal of Art Therapy 19,* 3–9.

Lambert, K. (2008) *Lifting Depression: A Neuroscientist's Hands-on Approach.* New York: Basic Books.

Landgarten, H.B. (1987) *Family Art Psychotherapy.* New York: Brunner/Mazel.

LaPierre, J. (2016) 'AA for Atheists: How to Take What You Need and Leave the Rest.' Available at www.choosehelp.com/topics/alcoholism/aa-for-atheists-2013-how-to-take-what-you-need-and-leave-the-rest, accessed on November 6, 2016.

Laurer, M. and van der Vennet, R. (2015) 'Effect of art production on negative mood and anxiety for adults in treatment for substance abuse.' *Art Therapy* 32, 4, 177–183.

Leonard, L.S. (1990) *Witness to the Fire: Creativity and the Veil of Addiction.* Boston, MA: Shambhala.

Levine, S. (1992) *Poiesis: The Language of Psychology and the Speech of the Soul.* London: Jessica Kingsley Publishers.

Liebmann, M. (2004) *Art Therapy for Groups: A Handbook of Themes and Exercises.* New York: Routledge (original work published 1986).

Loneck, B., Garrett, J.A., and Banks, S.M. (1996) 'A comparison of the Johnson Intervention with four other methods of referral to outpatient treatment.' *American Journal of Alcohol Abuse* 22, 2, 233–246.

Lounsbury, L. (2015, July) 'A Media Properties Continuum for Art Therapy in Substance Use Disorder Recovery.' Paper presented at the annual conference of the American Art Therapy Association (AATA), Minneapolis, MN.

Lovell, S. (2001) 'Loving Body is Embracing Spirit.' In M. Farrelly-Hansen (ed.) *Spirituality and Art Therapy* (pp.182–203). London: Jessica Kingsley Publishers.

Lowenfeld, V. and Brittain, W.L. (1987) *Creative and Mental Growth.* Upper Saddle River, NJ: Prentice-Hall (original work published 1947).

Luzzatto, P. (1987) 'The internal world of drug-abusers.' *British Journal of Projective Psychology* 32, 2, 22–33.

Luzzatto, P. (1989) 'Drinking Problems and Short-term Art Therapy.' In A. Gilroy and T. Dalley (eds) *Pictures at an Exhibition: Selected Essays on Art and Art Therapy* (pp.207–219). London: Routledge.

Mahony, J. (1999) 'Art Therapy and Art Activities in Alcohol Services.' In D. Waller and J. Mahony (eds) *Treatment of Addiction: Current Issues for Arts Therapies* (pp.117–140). London: Routledge.

Mahony, J. and Waller, D. (1992) 'Art Therapy in the Treatment of Alcohol and Drug Abuse.' In D. Waller and A. Gilroy (eds) *Art Therapy: A Handbook* (pp.172–188). Buckingham: Open University Press.

Manley, S. (2014, July) 'Anxiety Reduction During Detoxification Via Art Therapy Interventions.' Paper presented at the annual conference of the American Art Therapy Association (AATA), San Antonio, TX.

Martin, J. (1972) 'Chalk Talk on Alcohol' [video]. Havre de Grace, MD: Ashley Addiction Treatment.

Matto, H.C. (1997) 'An integrative approach to the treatment of women with eating disorders.' *The Arts in Psychotherapy* 24, 347–354.

Matto, H.C. (2002) 'Integrating art therapy methodology in brief inpatient substance abuse treatment for adults.' *Journal of Social Work Practice in the Addictions 2*, 2, 69–83.

Matto, H., Corcoran, J., and Fassler, A. (2003) 'Integrating solution-focused and art therapies for substance abuse treatment.' *The Arts in Psychotherapy 30*, 265–272.

McCauley, K. (2009) 'Pleasure Unwoven' [video]. Salt Lake City, UT: Institute for Addiction Study.

McClean, C. (1999) 'Mixed Metaphors—Dependency or Defence.' In D. Waller and J. Mahony (eds) *Treatment of Addiction: Current Issues for Arts Therapies* (pp.167–206). London: Routledge.

McCollum, E.E. and Trepper, T.S. (2001) *Family Solutions for Substance Abuse*. New York: Haworth.

McLachlan, J.F.C. and Head, V.B. (1974) 'An impairment rating scale for human figure drawings.' *Journal of Clinical Psychology 30*, 3, 405–407.

McNeilly, G. (2006) *Group Analytic Art Therapy*. London: Jessica Kingsley Publishers.

Mendenhall, A. (2014) 'Beyond opiates.' *Advances in Addiction and Recovery 2*, 1, 23–26.

Meyers, R.J., Miller, W.R., Hill, D.E., and Tonigan J.S. (1999) 'Community Reinforcement and Family Training (CRAFT): Engaging unmotivated drug users through concerned significant others.' *Journal of Substance Abuse 10*, 3, 291–308.

Miller, W.R. and Rollnick, S. (2013) *Motivational Interviewing: Helping People Change*. New York: Guilford Press (original work published 1991).

Mills, A. (2015) *Diagnostic Drawing Series Resource List*. Available at www.diagnosticdrawingseries.com/resource.pdf, accessed on January 7, 2015.

Milne, L.C. and Greenway, P. (2001) 'Drawings and defense style in adults.' *The Arts in Psychotherapy 28*, 245–249.

Minuchin, S. (1993) *Family Healing*. New York: Macmillan.

Moon, B. (2007) 'Dialoguing with dreams in existential art therapy.' *Art Therapy 24*, 3, 128–133.

Mooney, A.J., Dold, C., and Eisenberg, H. (2014) *The Recovery Book*. New York: Workman (original work published 1992).

Moore, R.W. (1983) 'Art therapy with substance abusers: A review of the literature.' *The Arts in Psychotherapy 10*, 251–260.

Morse, N., Thomson, L.J.M., Brown, Z., and Chatterjee, H. (2015) 'Effects of creative museum outreach sessions on measures of confidence, sociability and well-being for mental health and addiction recovery service-users.' *Arts and Health 7*, 3, 231–246.

Moschini, L.B. (2005) *Drawing the Line: Art Therapy with the Difficult Client*. Hoboken, NJ: Wiley.

NAADAC, The Association for Addiction Professionals (2016 rev.) *NAADAC Code of Ethics*. Available at www.naadac.org/code-of-ethics, accessed on January 19, 2017.

Naitove, C.E. (1976) 'Symbolic patterns in drawings by habitual users of street drugs.' *Confinia Psychiatrica 21*, 112–118.

NCADD (National Council on Alcoholism and Drug Dependence) (2015, June 27) 'Alcohol Energy Drinks.' Available at www.ncadd.org/about-addiction/alcohol/alcohol-energy-drinks, accessed on January 5, 2017.

NIDA (National Institute on Drug Abuse) (2012) *Principles of Drug Addiction Treatment: A Research-based Guide.* Washington, DC: NIDA.

NIDA (2013) *Marijuana Facts for Teens.* Available at www.drugabuse.gov/sites/default/files/teens_brochure_2013.pdf, accessed on May 7, 2015.

NIDA (2015) *Drugs, Brains, and Behavior: The Science of Addiction.* Washington, DC: NIDA.

Nobis, W. (2010) *The Art of Recovery: A Reflective and Creative Path Through the Twelve Steps.* Mustang, OK: Tate.

Nuckols, C.C. (2016, June) 'The 12 Steps and Beyond.' Paper presented at the NAADAC Behavioral Health Conference, Lincoln, NE.

Palmer, G. (2014) 'Motivational interviewing in art therapy.' *Art Therapy 31*, 3, 137–138.

Partnership News Service (2016) 'Powerful Heroin Substitute Called Pink Being Sold Online.' Available at www.drugfree.org/news-service/powerful-heroin-substitute-called-pink-sold-online, accessed on October 30, 2016.

Perkoulidis, S.A. (2009) 'Multifamily Group Art Therapy for Adolescent Substance Abuse.' In S.L. Brooke (ed.) *The Use of Creative Therapies with Chemical Dependency Issues* (pp.69–79). Springfield, IL: Charles C. Thomas.

Prochaska, J., DiClemente, C., and Norcross, J. (1992) 'In search of how people change: Applications to addictive behaviors.' *American Psychologist 47*, 9, 1002–1114.

Ranganathan, S. and Malick, R. (2013) 'Art-based Therapies for Substance Users and Their Families.' In P. Howie, S. Prasad, and J. Kristel (eds) *Using Art Therapy with Diverse Populations: Crossing Cultures and Abilities* (pp.225–233). London: Jessica Kingsley Publishers.

Riley, S. (1999a) *Contemporary Art Therapy with Adolescents.* London: Jessica Kingsley Publishers.

Riley, S. (1999b) 'Brief therapy: An adolescent invention.' *Art Therapy 16*, 2, 83–86.

Riley, S. (ed.) (2001) *Group Process Made Visible: Group Art Therapy.* Philadelphia, PA: Brunner-Routledge.

Rockwell, P. and Dunham, M. (2006) 'The utility of the Formal Elements Art Therapy Scale in assessment for substance use disorder.' *Art Therapy 23*, 3, 104–111.

Rohr, R. (2011) *Breathing Under Water: Spirituality and the Twelve Steps.* Cincinnati, OH: Franciscan Media.

Rohr, R. (2015) *Healing Images.* Center for Action and Contemplation. Available at www.cac.org/category/daily-meditations, accessed on October 14, 2015.

Rosal, M. (2016) 'Cognitive-Behavioral Art Therapy.' In J.A. Rubin (ed.) *Approaches to Art Therapy: Theory and Technique* (pp.333–352). New York: Routledge (original work published 1987).

Rubin, J.A. (2005) *Artful Therapy*. Hoboken, NJ: Wiley.

Rubin, J.A. (2011) *The Art of Art Therapy*. New York: Routledge (original work published 1984).

SAMHSA (Substance Abuse and Mental Health Services Administration) (2008) *Substance Abuse and Suicide Prevention* (white paper). Rockville, MD: SAMHSA.

SAMHSA (2016) 'Reports and Detailed Tables from the 2015 National Survey on Drug Use and Health.' Available at www.samhsa.gov/samhsa-data-outcomes-quality/major-data-collections/reports-detailed-tables-2015-NSDUH, accessed on July 15, 2016.

Schmanke, L. (2005, November) 'Bridges to Recovery.' Paper presented at the Annual Conference of the American Art Therapy Association (AATA), Atlanta, GA.

Schmanke, L. (2006, November) 'Harnessing the Power of Imagery to Rebuild Women's Lives.' Paper presented at the Annual Conference of the American Art Therapy Association (AATA), New Orleans, LA.

Schmanke, L. (2015, July) 'Escape from the Negativity Quagmire: Bridging Terrains with Adolescents.' Paper presented at the Annual Conference of the American Art Therapy Association (AATA), Minneapolis, MN.

Schmanke, L. (2016) 'Art Therapy and Substance Abuse.' In D.E. Gussak and M.L. Rosal (eds) *The Wiley Handbook of Art Therapy* (pp.361–374). Chichester: John Wiley & Sons.

Scott, E.H. and Ross, C.J. (2006) 'Integrating the creative arts into trauma and addiction treatment: Eight essential processes.' *Journal of Chemical Dependency Treatment 8*, 2, 207–226.

Siporin, S. (2010) 'Addicts to artists: The "good enough mother" in the substance abuse clinic.' *Psychodynamic Practice 16*, 3, 323–329.

Skaife, S. and Huet, V. (1998) 'Dissonance and Harmony: Theoretical Issues in Art Psychotherapy Groups.' In S. Skaife and V. Huet (eds) *Art Psychotherapy Groups: Between Pictures and Words* (pp.17–43). London: Routledge.

Skeffington, P.M. and Browne, M. (2014) 'Art therapy, trauma, and substance misuse: Using imagery to explore a difficult past with a complex client.' *International Journal of Art Therapy 19*, 3, 114–121.

Smith, R.L. (2013) 'Major Substances of Abuse and the Body.' In P.W. Stevens and R.L. Smith (eds) *Substance Abuse Counseling: Theory and Practice* (5th edn) (pp.51–97). Upper Saddle River, NJ: Pearson Education.

Speert, D. (2016) *Eco-Art Therapy: Deepening Connections with the Natural World*. American Art Therapy Association. Available at http://multibriefs.com/briefs/aata/ecoart102716.pdf, accessed on January 10, 2017.

Spring, D. (1985) 'Symbolic language of sexually abused, chemically dependent women.' *American Journal of Art Therapy 24*, 13–21.

Springham, N. (1992, Spring) 'Short-term group processes in art therapy for people with substance misuse problems.' *Inscape* 8–16.

Springham, N. (1998) 'The Magpie's Eye: Patients' Resistance to Engagement in an Art Therapy Group for Drug and Alcohol Patients.' In S. Skaife and V. Huet (eds) *Art Psychotherapy Groups: Between Pictures and Words* (pp.133–155). London: Routledge.

Springham, N. (1999) '"All Things Very Lovely": Art Therapy in a Drug and Alcohol Treatment Programme.' In D. Waller and J. Mahony (eds) *Treatment of Addiction: Current Issues for Arts Therapies* (pp.141–166). London: Routledge.

Stevens, P.W. and Smith, R.L. (eds) (2013) *Substance Abuse Counseling: Theory and Practice* (5th edn). Upper Saddle River, NJ: Pearson Education (original work published 1998).

Streetdrugs.org (2016) *Streetdrugs: Annual Drug Identification Guide*. Berkeley, CA: Publishers Group West.

Tait, C. (2013) 'Working with Special Populations.' In P.W. Stevens and R.L. Smith (eds) *Substance Abuse Counseling: Theory and Practice* (5th edn) (pp.287–310). Upper Saddle River, NJ: Pearson Education.

Teasdale, C. (1993, Summer) 'Filling time and space: Art therapy in the treatment of persistent alcohol misuse.' *Inscape* 17–23.

Trafton, J.A. (2015) *Understanding Substance-related and Addictive Disorders: Diagnosis, Treatment, and Prevention* (Supplement to training session). Los Banos, CA: Institute for Brain Potential.

Trafton, J.A. and Gifford, E.R. (2008) 'Behavioral reactivity and addiction: The adaptation of behavioral response to reward opportunities.' *Journal of Neuropsychiatry and Clinical Neurosciences 20*, 1, 23–35.

Turner, N., Welches, P., and Conti, S. (2013) *Mindfulness-based Sobriety*. Oakland, CA: New Harbinger.

Ulman, E. (1953) 'Art therapy at an outpatient clinic.' *Psychiatry 16*, 55–64.

Verinis, J.S., Lichtenberg, E.F., and Henrich, L. (1974) 'The Draw-a-Person in the Rain technique: Its relationship to diagnostic category and other personality indicators.' *Journal of Clinical Psychology 30*, 3, 407–414.

Virshup, E. (1985) 'Group art therapy in a methadone clinic lobby.' *Journal of Substance Abuse Treatment 2*, 153–158.

Wadeson, H.C. (2000) *Art Therapy Practice: Innovative Approaches with Diverse Populations*. New York: Wiley.

Wadeson, H. (2010) *Art Psychotherapy*. Hoboken, NJ: Wiley (original work published 1980).

Walitzer, K.S., Dermen, K.H., and Connors, G.J. (1999) 'Strategies for preparing clients for treatment.' *Behavior Modification 23*, 129–151.

Waller, D. (1993) *Group Interactive Art Therapy: Its Use in Training and Treatment*. London: Routledge.

Waller, D. and Mahony, J. (eds) (1999) *Treatment of Addiction: Current Issues for Arts Therapies*. London: Routledge.

Wegscheider-Cruse, S. (1989) *Another Chance: Hope and Health for the Alcoholic Family*. Palo Alto, CA: Science and Behavior Books (original work published 1981).

Wegscheider-Cruse, S. (1991) *The Family Trap*. Rapid City, SD: Onsite Training (original work published by Johnson Institute, 1976).

Weiser, J. (1999) *PhotoTherapy Techniques*. Vancouver, BC: PhotoTherapy Centre (original work published by Jossey-Bass, 1993).

White, W.L. (2014) 'Spirituality and addiction recovery: An interview with Ernie Kurtz, PhD.' *Advances in Addiction and Recovery 2*, 4, 22–29.

Wilkinson, R.A. and Chilton, G. (2013) 'Positive art therapy: Linking positive psychology to art therapy theory, practice, and research.' *Art Therapy 30*, 1, 4–11.

Willey, D. (2016) *Substance Use Disorders: Diagnosis and Treatment* (Supplement to training session). Olathe, KS: Cottonwood Springs Behavioral Health.

Willis, L.R., Joy, S.P., and Kaiser, D.H. (2010) 'Draw-a-Person-in-the-Rain as an assessment of stress and coping resources.' *The Arts in Psychotherapy 37*, 233–239.

Wilson, M. (2012) 'Art Therapy in Addictions Treatment: Creativity and Shame Reduction.' In C.A. Malchiodi (ed.) *Handbook of Art Therapy* (pp.302–319). New York: Guilford Press (original work published 2002).

Winnicott, D.W. (2005) *Playing and Reality*. London: Routledge (original work published 1971).

Winship, G. (1999) 'Group Therapy in the Treatment of Drug Addiction.' In D. Waller and J. Mahony (eds) *Treatment of Addiction* (pp.46–58). London: Routledge.

Wise, S. (2009) 'Extending a Hand: Open Studio Art Therapy in a Harm Reduction Center.' In S.L. Brooke (ed.) *The Use of Creative Therapies with Chemical Dependency Issues* (pp.37–50). Springfield, IL: Charles C. Thomas.

Wittenberg, D. (1975) 'Art Therapy for Adolescent Substance Abusers.' In E. Ulman and P. Dachinger (eds) *Art Therapy in Theory and Practice* (pp.150–158). New York: Schocken Books.

Woititz, J.G. (1990) *Adult Children of Alcoholics*. Deerfield, FL: Health Communications (original work published 1983).

Woodford, M.S. (2012) *Men, Addiction, and Intimacy: Strengthening Recovery by Fostering the Emotional Development of Boys and Men*. New York: Routledge.

Woods, A. and Springham, N. (2011) 'On learning from being the in-patient.' *International Journal of Art Therapy 16*, 2, 60–68.

Wu, N.S., Schairer, L.C., Dellor, D., and Grella, C. (2010) 'Childhood trauma and health outcomes in adults with comorbid substance abuse and mental health disorders.' *Addictive Behavior 35*, 1, 68–71.

Yalom, I.D. (2009) *The Gift of Therapy*. New York: HarperCollins (original work published 2002).

Yalom, I.D., with Leszcz, M. (2005) *The Theory and Practice of Group Psychotherapy*. Cambridge, MA: Basic Books (original work published Yalom 1970).

Author Note

Libby Schmanke, MS, board-certified art therapist (ATR-BC) and faculty member at Emporia State University's graduate art therapy program for 15 years, has presented regularly about art therapy and substance abuse at regional and national conferences, and has served for over 12 years for the Art Therapy Credentials Board. A licensed clinical addictions counselor (LCAC) with 25 years' experience in a variety of settings, she also holds the national Master Addiction Counselor (MAC) credential. She can be reached at eschmank@emporia.edu

Subject Index

Al 173–2
  group islands task 177–9
  refreshed treatment approach 177
  RRR process with Al's bridge drawing 174–6
Abstinence Violation Effect (AVE) 66
Acceptance and Commitment Therapy (ACT) 155
acceptance of paradox 158–9
acronyms 20–1
activities 211
  assertiveness continuum and storyboard 214–15
  biopsychosocial-spiritual (BPSS) "pie" 211–13
  emotional regulation through activities 140–1
  family forest task 224–6
  group activities to enhance cohesion 124–8
  mapping triggers and creating a trigger-safe environment 219–21
  mountaintop self-portrait 215–17
  Replication, Re-vision, and Reflection (RRR) 223–4
  themes for paper wall quilts 217–19
  your inner critic 222
addiction 43–4, 158
  addiction counseling 17–19
  Addiction Severity Index (ASI) 87
  brain function 44–6
  pharmaceutical approaches to treatment 46–7
ADDRESSING model directive 171–2
adolescents 170, 179
  adolescent group work 186–7
  Brandon's group 187–9, 189–90
  combined theoretical approaches in art therapy treatment 183–4
  etiology of adolescent substance abuse 181–2
  importance of the holding environment 189–90
  individual work with adolescents 184–5
  normal developmental issues 180–1
  resilience 182–3
  resistance 182
  Suzanne 185–6
Adult Children of Alcoholics 195, 198–9
Adverse Childhood Experiences (ACEs) 142, 143, 181
aesthetic art activities 156–7
agonist drug treatments 46
Al-Anon 195, 198
alcohol 54
  alcoholic energy drinks (AEDs) 56
Alcohol and Drug Abuse Primary Treatment (ADAPT) program 10-13
Alcohol Information School 112
Alcoholics Anonymous World Service (AAWS) 164
Alcoholics Anonymous® (AA) 18, 45, 46, 145, 150, 155, 198
  spirituality 162–3
  Twelve Steps model 63–4
alcoholism 43–4
American Medical Association (AMA) 43
amusement park technique 34, 99, 101–2
anger 132
anhedonia 47, 56, 58
Ann's bridge drawing 137–8
antagonist drug treatments 46–7
anxiety 37, 135–6
archetypal themes 38–40
Aristotle 151
art psychotherapy 12

art therapy 11, 16, 17–19
  adolescents 183–4
  benefits 41
  and cognitive behavioral therapy (CBT) 66–7
  family art therapy with addiction issues 200–4
  group activities to enhance cohesion 124–8
  group models 110–11
  incorporating art therapy into substance abuse treatment 25–7
  and nature 154–5
  and neuroscience 47–51
Art Therapy Credentials Board (ATCB) Code of Ethics 170
assertiveness work 115–17, 214–15
assessment 31–2, 87, 108
  and diagnosis 87–8
  common themes and symbols 32–4, 90–3
  contributions of informal art assessment 88–9
  formal and informal projective assessment 94–8
  metaphorical and projective drawing tasks 34, 99–108
  research on drawing assessment 89–90
attachment 142–3, 144–5
Ault, Marilyn 15–16
Ault, Robert 9, 16

Beattie, Melody *(Codependent No More)* 191
biopsychosocial (BPS) model 43, 44, 51–3, 204
biopsychosocial-spiritual (BPSS) model 51
  art activity 211–13
  handout for clients 213–14
Bird's Nest Drawing (BND) 22, 31, 34, 89, 99
Black, Claudia 191
body maps 137
Boughn, Alison 226
Bradshaw, John *(Healing the Shame that Binds You)* 191
brain function 44–7
  art therapy and neuroscience 47–51
Brandon 187–9, 189–90
Brandt, Samantha 156
bridge drawing 28, 34, 59–60, 72, 89, 99, 102–4, 105, 223
  Ann's bridge drawing 137–8
  Jerry's bridge drawing 95–6
  Judy and Marissa 120–1
  labeling 106–8
  prognostication 97–8
  RRR process with Al's bridge drawing 174–6
Buddhism 155

caffeinated alcoholic beverages (CABs) 56
case materials 19
  Al 173–9
  Ann's bridge drawing 137–8
  Brandon's group 187–9, 189–90
  Heidi 49–51, 91, 146–8
  Irene 9–15
  Jay 115–17
  Jerry's bridge drawing 95–6
  Josie 71–2
  Judy and Marissa 120–1
  Manyara's group 122–3
  Marquette 92–3
  Martha 74–85
  Richard 92
  Rick's "Amazing Grace" 152–3
  Suzanne 185–6
  Teresa 132–5
  Wilson family 204–11
Centers for Disease Control and Prevention (CDC) 142
children, roles of 195–7
  adult children 197
client resistance 162–3
  adolescents 182
cocaine 57–8
Cocaine Anonymous 63, 164
codependency 191–2
  dynamics of 193–5
cognitive behavioral therapy (CBT) 65, 133
  art therapy and 66–7
  locus of control 65–6
collage 11–15
Community Reinforcement and Family Training (CRAFT) 200
control 65–6
Controlled Substances Act (US) 61
counseling 10–11
creative arts therapies 30–1
crisis directive 27, 99
cultural considerations 170
  ADDRESSING model directive 171–2
  Replication, Re-vision, and Reflection (RRR) technique 172–3

Department of Corrections 10
depressants 53–4
designer drugs 61
detoxification 28
developmental issues 36
diagnosis 87–8
  contributions of informal art assessment 88–9
Diagnostic and Statistical Manual of Mental Disorders, 5th Edition (DSM-5) 20, 87–8
Diagnostic Drawing Series (DDS) 94

Dialectic Behavior Therapy (DBT) 155
disease, addiction as 43–4
diversity 170
  AI 173–9
  cultural considerations 170–3
dopamine 44–6, 51, 56, 144–5
Draw a Person in the Rain (DAPR) 34, 99
dream work 154
Drug Enforcement Agency 61
drugs of abuse 53
  alcohol and other sedatives 54
  depressants 53–4
  legal and treatment issues with new drugs 61
  opioids 55
  stimulants 56–60

embedded family groups 199–200
enabling behavior 193–4
existential themes 38–40
expressive arts therapies 30–1
Expressive Therapies Continuum (ETC) 22, 35–6, 43, 48, 94

false self 118–19
family therapy 29–30, 191
  adult children 197
  combined approaches 200
  dynamics of codependency 193–5
  embedded family groups 199–200
  family art therapy with addiction issues 200–4
  family forest task 210, 224–6
  family rules 192–3
  family theory pertaining to addictions 191–2
  intervention 199
  roles typical of children 195–7
  self-help groups 198–9
  standard treatment approaches 198–200
  Wilson family 204–11
fear 135–6
feelings 37, 129
  addressing negative feelings 131–9
  approaches to feelings work 130–1
  benefits of art therapy 148–9
  body maps 137
  feelings-monster task 132–5
  positive approaches 139–41
First Step Series 27, 99
flow state 140–1
Food and Drug Administration (FDA) 58
Formal Elements Art Therapy Scale (FEATS) 31–2, 89, 94

graduation walls 125–6
gratitude 160–1
grief 136–7
group islands task 177–9
group therapy 10, 34–5, 109
  adolescent group work 186–7
  art therapy group models 110–11
  benefits of group work 109–10
  group activities to enhance cohesion 124–8
  group imagery 119–21
  group member roles 123–4
  Manyara's group 122–3
  Motivational Interviewing (MI) and Stages of Change (SOC) approach 111–18
  narcissism and the false self 118–19
  therapist's role 121–2

harm reduction 29
Heidi 49–51, 91, 146–8
heroin 46, 55, 61
holding environment 142–3, 189–90
holistic approaches 30
hospital-based settings 28
humility 160

illustrations 19
imagery 118–19
  group 119–21
  transformative effects of 151–2
incident drawing 27, 35, 79, 80, 99
individual modality 72–3
  Rhoda 73–4
inner critic 139, 222
inspirational readings 153–4
interpretation of artwork 94–5
  Jerry's bridge drawing 95–6
  media 96
  prognostication and hindsight 97–8
  red flags 96–7
intervention 199
Irene 9–15

Jay 115–17
jealousy 132–5
Jerry 95–6
Josie 71–2, 86
Judy 120

Kinetic Family Drawing (K-F-D) 32, 76–7, 99
Kinetic House-Tree-Person (K-H-T-P) drawing 76, 77–8, 79, 97, 99, 112–13, 185, 188, 203, 223

labeling 106–8
Ladder of Change 36
legal issues 61
loss 136–7

Manyara 122–3
marijuana 58–60
Marissa 120–1
Marquette 92–3
Martha 74–5, 84–5, 86, 130
 art impressions 76–8, 79–80, 81–4
 goals and assessment 76, 78–9, 80–1
maturity issues 36
media 96
metaphorical drawing tasks, 34 99–100
 amusement park technique 101–2
 Draw a Person in the Rain (DAPR) 100–1
 labeling 106–8
 paper spanning 105
 road drawings 100
 vertical orientation 105–6
methamphetamine 56–7
mindfulness 155–6
Mindfulness-based Relapse Prevention (MBRP) 155
Minnesota model 64
Motivational Interviewing (MI) and the Stages of Change (SOC) 22, 27–8, 67–9, 73, 99, 110, 111–12, 183, 185, 200–1
 historical support for MI/SOC in addiction treatment 69–71
 Jay 115–17
 Josie 71–2
 model for action stage interactive groups 113–15
 screening methods and 112–13
mountaintop self-portrait 118–19, 215–17

Nar-Anon 195, 198
Narateen 198
narcissism 118–19
Narcotics Anonymous® (NA) 18, 63, 81, 150, 162–3, 164
natural world 154–5
negative feelings 131–2
 anger 132
 Ann's bridge drawing 137–8
 fear and anxiety 135–6
 grief and loss 136–7
 jealousy 132–5
 shame 139
neuroscience 43
 art therapy and neuroscience 47–51
Niebuhr, Reinhold 159

open-mindedness 160
opioids 55
Overeaters Anonymous 63
oxytocin 60, 144

paper spanning 105
paper wall quilts 125
 themes for 217–19
paradox 158–9
parole 9–10, 12, 13
Person Picking an Apple from a Tree (PPAT) 32
pharmaceutical approaches to treatment 46–7
PhotoTherapy 201–2
positive feelings 139–40
 emotional regulation through activities 140–1
post-traumatic stress disorder (PTSD) 43, 47, 49, 129, 145
 impact of childhood trauma on adult PTSD 141–2
powerlessness 159
prescription painkillers 55
prison sentences 9–10
 after release 12
projective drawings 34, 94, 99–100
 amusement park technique 101–2
 bridge drawings 102–4
 Draw a Person in the Rain (DAPR) 100–1
 interpretation 94–5
 interpreter projection 95–6
 labeling 106–8
 media 96
 paper spanning 105
 prognostication and hindsight 97–8
 red flags 96–7
 road drawings 100
 vertical orientation 105–6
prostitution 9, 10
psychodynamically informed approaches 23–5
psychoeducation 64–5

rape 13, 15, 54, 145
Rational Emotive Behavior Therapy (REBT) 65, 130–1
 reframing directive for REBT 131
recovery 158, 194
 acceptance of paradox 158–9
 client resistance 162–3
 gratitude 160–1
 open-mindedness and humility 160
 powerlessness and transformation 159
 religion 161–2
red flags 96–7

relapse triggers 12, 75, 80, 81, 125, 136, 138
  mapping triggers and creating a trigger-safe environment 219–21
  paper wall quilt theme 218–19
relationships 143, 144–5
religion 161–2, 168–9
Replication, Re-vision, and Reflection (RRR) technique 172–3, 223
  caveats 224
  client and client's drawing 223
  performing the RRR 223
  RRR process with Al's bridge drawing 174–6
resilience 182–3
Rhoda 73–4, 85
Richard 92
Rick 152–3
road drawing 34, 89, 99, 100
role-play with masks 115–17

Satir, Virginia 191, 195, 203
scapegoating 35, 121, 203
  children 194, 197, 201, 206, 210
sedatives 54
Self Image directive 25
self-help groups 198–9
self-portrait flag line 126–8
Sex Addicts Anonymous 63
sexual issues 143–5
shame 37–8, 139
  inner critic 139, 222
Silkworth, William 43
Skinner, B.F. 164
solution-focused therapy 29
spirituality 38–40, 150, 168–9
  and addiction 150–1
  aesthetic art activities 156–7
  biopsychosocial-spiritual (BPSS) model 51, 211–14
  dream work 154
  inspirational readings 153–4
  mindfulness 155–6
  nature and art therapy 154–5
  Rick's "Amazing Grace" 152–3
  special topics in addiction spirituality 158–63
  transformative effects of images 151–2
  Twelve Steps 164–8
Stages of Change (SOC) 22, 27–8, 36, 67–72
  action 69
  contemplation 68
  group therapy 111–17
  maintenance 69
  precontemplation 68

preparation 68
termination 69
Stages of Change Readiness and Treatment Eagerness Scale (SOCRATES) 27–8
steroids 60
stimulants 56
  cocaine 57–8
  marijuana 58–60
  methamphetamine 56–7
  other substances of abuse 60
Substance Abuse Subtle Screening Inventory (SASSI) 87
substance abuse theory 43, 62
  art therapy and neuroscience 47–51
  biopsychosocial model 51–3
  defining addiction 43–4
  drugs of abuse 53–60
  legal and treatment issues with new drugs 61
  substance abuse and brain function 44–7
substance abuse treatment 22, 41–2
  Alcoholics Anonymous and the Twelve Steps model 63–4
  assessment 31–4
  cognitive behavioral therapy (CBT) 65–7
  detoxification approach 28
  expressive and creative arts therapies 30–1
  factors in success 85–6
  family therapy 29–30
  group work 34–5
  harm reduction approach 29
  holistic approaches 30
  incorporating art therapy into 25–7
  individual modality 72–4
  Martha 74–85
  Minnesota model 64
  Motivational Interviewing (MI) and the Stages of Change (SOC) 27–8, 67–72
  psychodynamically informed approaches 23–5
  psychoeducation 64–5
  short-term hospital-based inpatient settings 28
  solution-focused therapy 29
  special topics for art therapy and addictions 35–8
  spiritual themes 38–40
  treatment approaches for families 198–200
  treatment for substance abuse and trauma 145–6
suicide 129, 138, 175, 211
Suzanne 185–6
symbols 32–4
symbols 90–1
  split faces 91–3

Teresa 132–5
terminology 19–20
themes 32–4, 90–1
  split faces 91–3
therapeutic relationship 182, 183–4
Tolkien, J.R.R. *(The Lord of the Rings)* 153–4
transformation 159
Transtheoretical Model (TTM) 22, 27
trauma 37–8, 129, 141
  attachment issues 142–3
  benefits of art therapy 148–9
  Heidi 146–8
  impact of childhood trauma on adult substance use 141–2
  sexual issues 143–5
  treatment for substance abuse and trauma 145–6
treatment romance 143, 144–5
triggers *see* relapse triggers
Twelve Steps 22, 36, 38, 40, 46, 63–4, 125, 139, 142, 150, 151, 153, 160, 162, 163, 165–168
spirituality 164–8
text of the Twelve Steps 165

US War on Drugs 10

vertical orientation 105–6

Wegscheider-Cruse, Sharon 191
Wilson family 204–6, 210
  initial art therapy session 206–8
  shifting of the identified patient 208–10
Wilson, Bill 43, 150, 198
Wilson, Lois 198
Woititz, Janet 191
Woodruff, Leslie 219–20
World Health Organization (WHO) 43

Author Index

AA (Alcoholics Anonymous) 43, 70, 159, 164, 165
Adedoyin, C. 30
Adelman, E. 30
Albert-Puleo, N. 23, 24, 32
Alberts, A. 181
Aletraris, L. 30
Allen, P. 26, 38, 156
Angheluta, A.M. 55
APA (American Psychiatric Association) 88
Arrington, D.B. 224–5
ASAM (American Society of Addiction Medicine) 44, 87
ATCB (Art Therapy Credentials Board, Inc.) 170
Ault, R.E. 33

Banks, S.M. 199
Barry, D. 66
Bellwood, L.R. 138
Biley, F.C. 31
Black, C. 192, 195, 202
Blos, P. 181
Booth, L. 161
Bowen, S. 155
Bowlby, J. 142
Breslin, K.T. 30
Bricker, M. 145
Brittain, W.L. 188
Brooke, S.L. 31
Brown, J. 141, 142
Browne, M. 35, 145
Burns, R.C. 94, 99

C., R. 164
Callaghan, G.M. 203
Cameron, J. 150

Canty, J. 119
Capuzzi, D. 45, 46
Carolan, R. 150–1, 181
Carr, R. 48
Castricone, L. 30
CDC (Centers for Disease Control and Prevention) 55
Chamberlain, L.L. 54
Chawla, N. 155
Chickerneo, N.B. 38
Chilton, G. 139–40, 140
Cicero, T.J. 55
Colgate, V. 38–9
Conger, D. 211
Connors, G.J. 67, 68, 113
Conti, S. 155
Corcoran, J. 29
Cox, K.L. 27, 35, 99
Crowe, A. 28
CSAT (Center for Substance Abuse Treatment) 73, 109
Csikszentmihalyi, M. 140

Deaver, S. 31, 89, 142
Dermen, K.H. 113
Devine, D. 32–3
Dickman, S.B. 32, 97
Dickson, C. 26
DiClemente, C. 27, 67
Diehls, V.A. 27–8
Dold, C. 44
Donnenberg, D. 34–5
Dore, E.A. 142
Dryden, W. 131
Dunham, M. 89
Dunn, J.E. 32
DuWors, G. 155

Eisenberg, H. 44
Elkind, D. 181
Ellis, A. 131
Emunah, R. 182
Engel, G.L. 51–2
Erdmann, G.W. 25
Erikson, E. 180

Fassler, A. 29
Faulkner, C.A. 44
Feen-Calligan, H. 28, 35, 156, 38, 40
Felitti, V.J. 142
Fernandez, K.M. 35
Flores, P.J. 142
Forrest, G. 37, 88
Fosha, D. 131
Foulke, W. 37
Francis, D. 31, 89
Fredrickson, B.L. 140
Furth, G.M. 106

Gantt, L.M. 31, 32
Garrett, J.A. 199
Gerber, N. 42
Gerity, L.A. 142
Gifford, E.R. 44–5, 45
Ginsberg, S. 181
Glidden, K. 141, 142
Glover, N.M. 38
Golomb, C. 96
Greenway, P. 90
Grof, C. 150
Groterath, A. 36
Groth-Marnat, G. 94
Gutman, S.A. 141

Hagens, C.A. 38
Haluzan, M. 30, 100
Hammer, E.F. 99, 100–1
Hanes, M.J. 34, 99, 100
Hanson, R. 139
Harms, E. 30–1
Hass-Cohen, N. 48
Hayes, P.M. 40
Hays, P.A. 171, 172
Hays, R.E. 28, 34, 99, 102, 103, 105, 106
Head, V.B. 30–1, 90
Heilig, M. 44
Henrich, L. 101
Hinz, L.D. 35–6, 48, 94, 97
Holt, E. 27, 32, 99, 103, 105
Horay, B.J. 27, 28
Horovitz, E.G. 38
Hoshino, J. 203
Hrenko, K.D. 34, 99, 101

Huet, V. 111, 119
Hull, A. 48

Inaba, D.S. 58, 59, 60

Johnson, D.R. 40
Johnson, J.L. 224
Johnson, L. 37, 139
Johnson, M.M. 171
Johnson, V. 199
Jones, C.M. 55
Joy, S.P. 34, 101
Julliard, K.N. 40
Jung, C.G. 150

Kagin, S.L. 35
Kaiser, D.H. 27, 31, 32, 34, 89, 99, 101, 103, 105, 142
Kasl, C.D. 143
Kaufman, G.H. 24–5, 34
Kaufman, S.H. 99
Keller, T. 37
Ketcham, K. 160
Khoury, L. 142
Korb, A. 160
Krebs, K.A. 40
Kuhn, C. 55, 60
Kurtz, E. 160, 162, 163

Lachman-Chapin, M. 24, 25
Lambert, K. 48
Landgarten, H.B. 202
LaPierre, J. 163
Laurer, M. 37
Lee, B.K. 55
Leonard, L.S. 150
Leszcz, M. 109, 112, 121
Levine, S. 151
Lichtenberg, E.F. 101
Liebmann, M. 118, 137
Loneck, B. 199
Lounsbury, L. 36
Lovell, S. 151
Lowenfeld, V. 188
Lusebrink, V.B. 35
Luzzatto, P. 25
Lyons, S. 28, 34, 99, 102, 103, 105, 106

Mahony, J. 22, 26, 31, 41
Malick, R. 29
Malone, S.B. 30
Manley, S. 37
Marlatt, A. 155
Martin, J. 70

AUTHOR INDEX

Matto, H.C. 28, 29, 36, 66, 67
McCauley, K. 44
McClean, C. 30
McCollum, E.E. 192, 203
McLachlan, J.F.C. 90
McNeilly, G. 119
Mendenhall, A. 46, 47
Meyers, R.J. 200
Miller, W.R. 27, 67, 68
Mills, A. 94
Milne, L.C. 90
Minuchin, S. 201, 203
Moon, B. 154
Mooney, A.J. 44, 46, 55, 144, 159, 162
Moore, R.W. 22, 33
Morse, N. 36
Moschini, L.B. 36
Moxley, D.P. 35

NAADAC (Association for Addiction Professionals) 87, 171
Naitove, C.E. 33
NCADD (National Council on Alcoholism and Drug Dependence) 55
NIDA (National Institute on Drug Abuse) 41, 44, 47, 59, 145
Nobis, W. 40
Norcross, J. 27
Nuckols, C.C. 46, 118

Osha, V. 24, 32

Palmer, G. 28
Parmenter, A.S. 28
Partnership News Service 61
Perkoulidis, S.A. 29
Petry, N.M. 66
Price, K. 27, 35, 99
Prochaska, J. 27, 67

Ranganathan, S. 29
Reed, M.R. 30
Riley, S. 110, 183, 184, 186
Rockwell, P. 89
Rohr, R. 151–2, 166
Rollnick, S. 27, 67, 68
Rosal, M. 66
Ross, C.J. 31, 137
Rubin, J.A. 23, 88

SAMHSA (Substance Abuse and Mental Health Services Administration) 55, 62, 129
Schindler, V.P. 141
Schmanke, L. 26, 98, 100, 105, 108, 180, 189

Scott, E.H. 31, 137
Siegel, D.J. 131
Siporin, S. 142
Skaife, S. 111, 119
Skeffington, P.M. 35, 145
Smith, R.L. 43, 54, 61, 63, 159, 199, 224
Solomon, M.F. 131
Speert, D. 154
Spring, D. 33, 145
Springham, N. 23, 23–4, 33, 34, 118, 119
Stauffer, M.D. 45, 46
Stevens, P.W. 43, 54, 63, 159, 199, 224
Streetdrugs.org 55, 58, 60, 61
Swartzwelder, S. 55

Tabone, C. 31
Tait, C. 181, 182
Teasdale, C. 33–4
Trafton, J.A. 44–5, 45, 46, 47
Trepper, T.S. 192, 203
Turner, N. 155

Ulman, E. 22

van der Vennet, R. 37
Verinis, J.S. 101
Virshup, E. 35

Wadeson, H.C. 26, 33, 100
Walitzer, K.S. 113
Waller, D. 22, 31, 110
Washington, O.G.M. 35
Wegscheider-Cruse, S. 195, 197
Weiser, J. 201
Welches, P. 155
White, W.L. 63, 163
Wilkinson, R.A. 139–40, 140
Willey, D. 47
Willis, L.R. 34, 101
Willis, R. 34, 99, 101
Wilson, M. 37, 139
Wilson, W. 55
Winnicott, D.W. 142–3, 189
Winship, G. 110
Wise, S. 29
Wittenberg, D. 34, 111
Woititz, J.G. 192, 197
Wolf, A. 32
Woodford, M.S. 131
Woods, A. 23
Wright, A.J. 94
Wu, N.S. 141

Yalom, I.D. 72, 112, 121, 154